D0928081

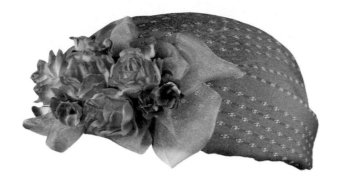

HATS

with values

Photography and Text by

Desire Smith

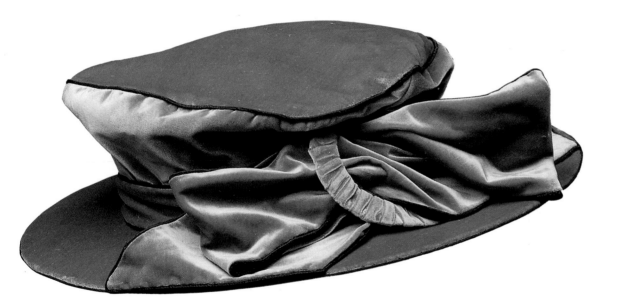

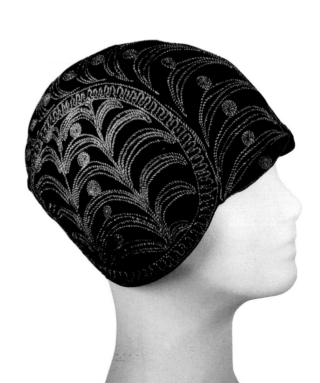

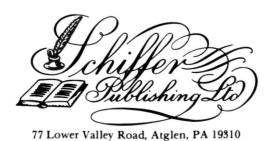

Schiffer Publishing Ltd

77 Lower Valley Road, Atglen, PA 19310

Dedicated to my husband, Bruce Smith

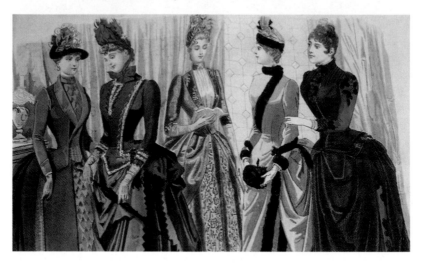

Library of Congress Cataloging-in-Publication Data

Smith, Desire.
    Hats / photography and text by Desire Smith.
        p.   cm.
    Includes bibliographical references and index.
    ISBN 0-7643-0030-X
    1. Hats--Collectors and collecting--United States--History--19th century. 2. Collectors and collecting--United States--History--20th century. 3. Vintage clothing--United States.
    I. Title
GT610.S63 1996
391.'43--dc20   96-7411
                                                      CIP

On the cover: Marcie Behanna, photographed by Desire Smith, wears a silk Edwardian dress with a ca. 1900 gray silk velvet hat with an overlay of black lace, embroidered in silk, with a floral design, additionally detailed with gray glass beads, trimmed with a white ostrich plume, lined with white silk and tulle; labeled Geo. Allen, Incorporated, 1214 Chestnut St., Philadelphia.

Title page: Contemporary hat, see p.141. Burnt orange hat, see p.94. Helmet style cloche, c.1920, decorated with metallic cord, labelled Gimbel Brothers, Philadelphia, Paris.

Published by Schiffer Publishing, Ltd.
77 Lower Valley Road
Atglen, PA 19310
Please write for a free catalog.
This book may be purchased from the publisher.
Please include $2.95 postage.
Try your bookstore first.

We are interested in hearing from authors
with book ideas on related subjects.

Contents

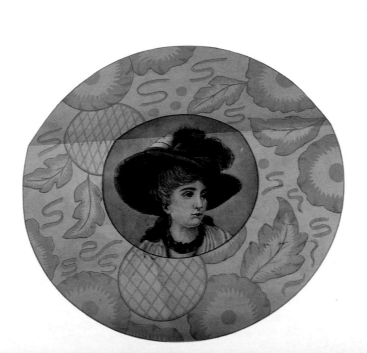

❦ Acknowledgments ❦

Sincere thanks to Peter and Nancy Schiffer for having the confidence to publish my book, and special thanks to Nancy for her patience with my numerous production questions. Also at Schiffer Publishing, thanks to Dawn Stoltzfus for her help in the creation of this book. Thanks to my husband, Bruce Smith for being a harsh critic, and to my sons, Matthew and Michael, for being enthusiastic. Thanks to Marcie Behanna for her time and patience as my hat model. You can judge a book by its cover!

A number of friends in the vintage clothing field deserve special mention. Elizabeth A. Freame, thanks for finding so many great hats for my collection; Alison Bartholomew (Petit Points, Millburn, New Jersey), and Karen Augusta (Antique Lace and Textiles, North Westminster, Vermont), thank you for trusting me to photograph your wonderful hats for the book. Donna Sigler (my former art teacher) thank you for your encouragement, and for giving me the Elizabeth Taylor straw. Sharon Glosser, Katherine Stauffer, Lois Fischer, and Edna Kandle, thank you for permitting me to photograph hats from your personal collections.

Dilys Blum, Curator of Costume and Textiles, Philadelphia Museum of Art, thank you for letting me peruse the files relating to Ahead of Fashion: Hats of the 20th Century, and for authorizing the use of photographs from the Bulletin relating to the exhibition. You have been an inspiration to all of us who love hats!

Bella Veksler, Curator of the Drexel Collection of Historic Fashion, thank you for permitting me to photograph a number of beautiful hats from the collection, and for sharing so freely your ideas and expertise relating to the millinery field, as well as your own wonderful designs, for the contemporary millinery chapter. Linda Eppich, Chief Curator, Rhode Island Historical Society, thank you for making my dream of having the Betsy Metcalf bonnet in the book reality.

Tabytha Campbell of Hats In the Belfry, thank you for your thoughtful interview. Claire Galicano, in Continuing Education, Elizabeth A. Plepis, and the talented millinery students at Moore College of Art, and especially Mr. Alzie, thank you for your patience with me, and for enhancing my book with your incredible hats.

Jay Foreman, thank you for taking time from your busy schedule to show me S & S Hats. It was a great learning experience for me, and I was thrilled to meet Don Anderson, one of my all-time favorite millinery designers.

Kelly Whalin of Wear It Again Sam and fashion designer, Louise Stewart, thank you for your friendship and enthusiasm; Barbara Consorto and Angela Grimes, my friends, thank you for trying to make me computer literate, you really tried, and Angela, thank you for spending countless hours with me at the computer.

✿ Preface ✿

Hats is about millinery—that is, women's hats, their design, history, and traditions. Hats is a picture book which explores the art of the hat. The hat is viewed as soft-sculpture, in an attempt to celebrate and delight in the craft of millinery, as well as to delineate styles, periods, and designers.

My purpose is to present a sampling of photographs which depict, by materials used and in chronological order, the best of the past in millinery and, in a final chapter, discuss the present and future for women's hats.

This is not a dirge for a cultural past when wearing hats was traditional and appropriate, but rather an acknowledgment of a grand and evolving tradition.

With a few additions from private collections, universities, and museums, the hats in this book were collected by the author. This is my collection, my passion, my obsession! Share with me the excitement. These are the days of hat collecting!

a dashing spirited line of hats...

buckram frames, smart,
silk velvet with ostrich feathers
over foundations of pasted flowers,
a dashing, spirited line of hats.

jaunty, upturned brims,
wing draped crowns, chic narrow brims,
grosgrain ribbon, rosettes,
cording, sweeping from back to front,
a dashing, spirited line of hats.

pearl drops, coquettish poke lines,
mushroom brims, tricornes,
taffeta, silk, peau de soie,
dull beads, cellophane wheels,
a dashing, spirited line of hats

fancy buckles, cotton duvetyne,
baronette satin, creased crowns,
bright feathers, brims that swoop
a dashing, spirited line of hats.

—Desire Smith

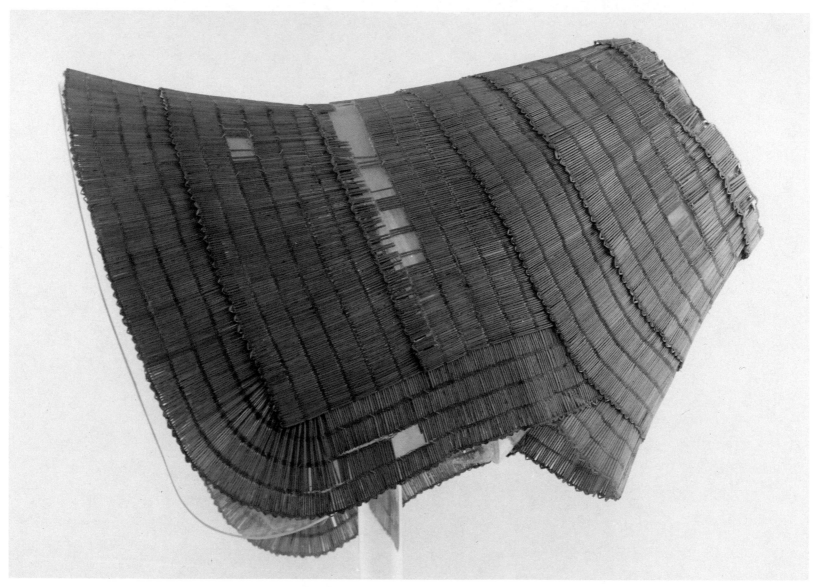

Metcalf bonnet. *Courtesy of The Rhode Island Historical Society.*

⟋ Straw ⟍

Natural straw used in millinery comes from dried stems of grains such as barley, oats, rye, and wheat. After the grain is pulled, it is laid on the ground and bleached. The outer layer of the stem is removed and the stem is bleached a second time. The straw is woven or plaited, either by hand or loom, then the braids are stitched together in a circular way to make a hat.

The highest quality straw used in making the early bonnets came from Leghorn, Italy, the English name for Livorno, Italy (Madeleine Ginsburg, *The Hat: Trends and Traditions*). When Americans began to fashion their own hats, they tried to find a straw as smooth and easy to work with as Leghorn.

Synthetic straw and the coating and treatment of natural straw to make it colorful and shiny was not commonplace until the 1950s. I do have several examples of 1930s and 1940s "cellophane" straw in my collection. Cellophane is a thin, transparent film made of acetate. Sometimes it is used over paper, but often it is used as ribbon-like strips to imitate straw.

The First Known American Straw Bonnet

Betsy Metcalf of Providence, Rhode Island, launched the American millinery industry on its way. At age twelve she made the first straw bonnet, described as Dunstable style, with a 5" brim of split straw, $\frac{1}{16}$" in diameter, slightly rounded on top, and laid parallel and stitched together at $\frac{3}{8}$" intervals, pleated at back, with center gather. The bonnet was given to the Rhode Island Historical Society in 1912 by Dr. Franklin C. Clark, Betsy's nephew.

Thanks to the efforts of Linda Eppich, Chief Curator at the Rhode Island Historical Society, the bonnet was photographed for publication here. This bonnet is an 1859 Betsy Metcalf Baker replica of her original, the first known American straw bonnet, which was made in 1798.

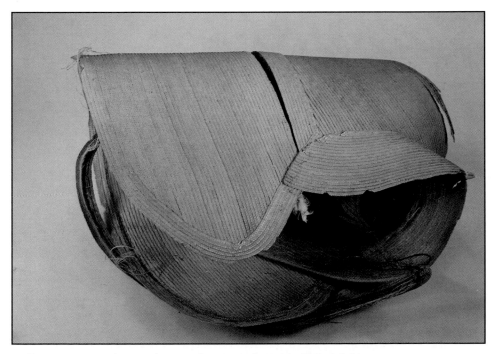

Ca. 1800 natural straw bonnet fragment, found in Philadelphia.

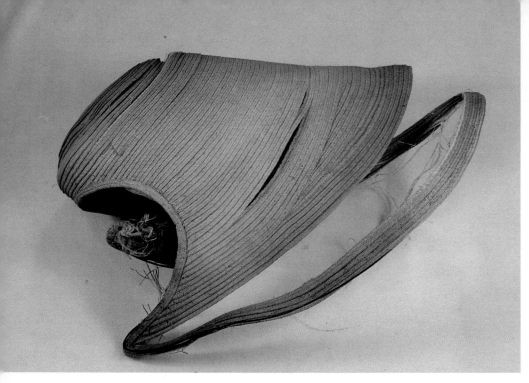

Ca. 1820 natural straw bonnet fragment.

Early American Bonnets

Early American bonnets have a special place in our history and culture that transcends fashion. These hats speak of a nation coming of age, discovering and using its native straw, fur, feathers, and wool. Recently independent, America was still looking to Europe for its inspiration in fashion!

The major cities supported an early and significant millinery trade, and as early as 1830 women of means had bonnets designed to match special outfits. The millinery trade steadily progressed until the Civil War. Certainly at that time, many clothing and hat makers turned

Ca. 1830 natural straw bonnet fragment, showing cotton lining.

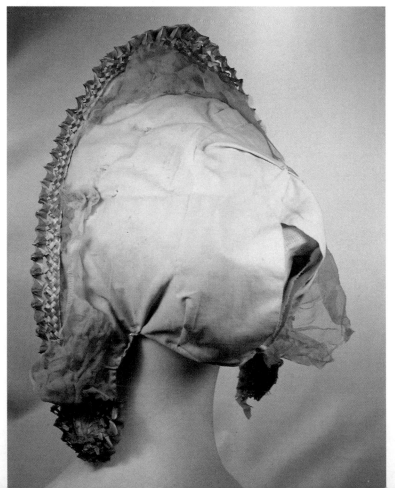

their efforts to the military. The millinery trade in the North was not as severely affected as it was in the South, where make-do and recycling in fashion was more common, due to the blockade.

However, the society of the time was preoccupied with the war effort, and social occasions, balls, and parties were not as well attended.

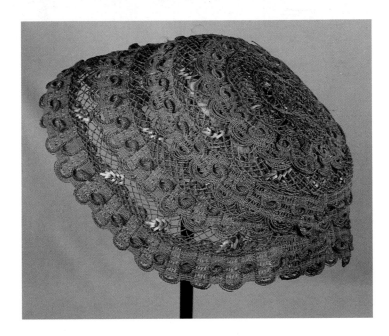

Ca. 1850 elaborately woven open-work natural straw bonnet, lined with pale blue silk; labeled Geo. W. Miles, Importer, 928 Chestnut St., Philada; Birkenbine Estate.

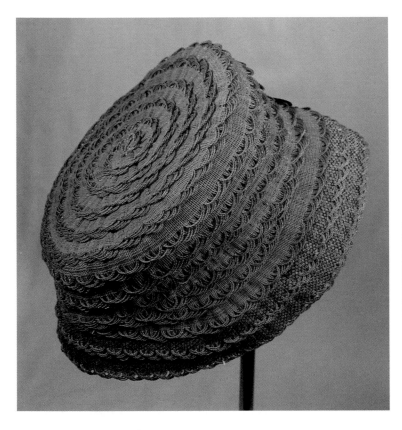

Ca. 1850 elaborately woven natural straw bonnet, trimmed with burgundy silk velvet, lined with silk; labeled Julius Sichel, 107 & 109 North Eighth St., Philada; Birkenbine Estate.

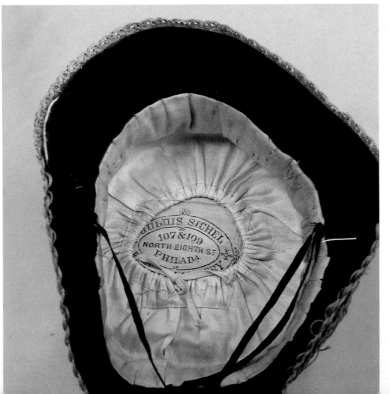

Inside view of ca. 1850 Sichel bonnet.

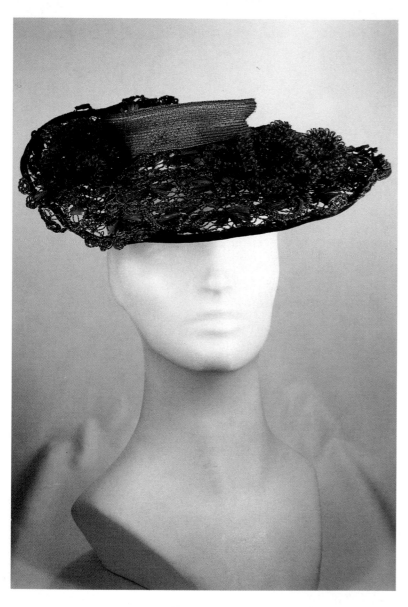

Ca. 1860 elaborately woven open-work, natural straw, lined with white silk.

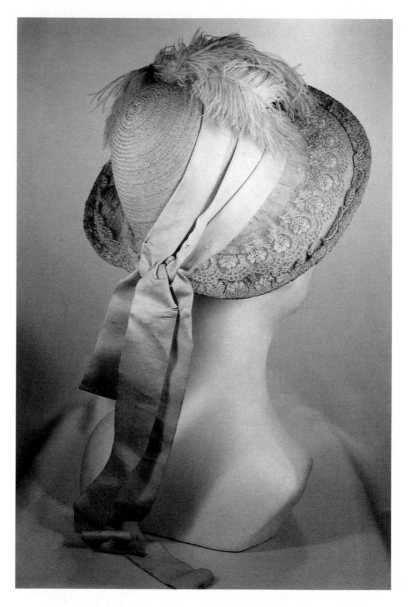

Ca. 1860 natural straw bonnet, trimmed with handmade lace, feathers, eggshell silk ribbon, and ruching; paper labeled showing three birds in flight. *Courtesy of Alison Bartholomew.*

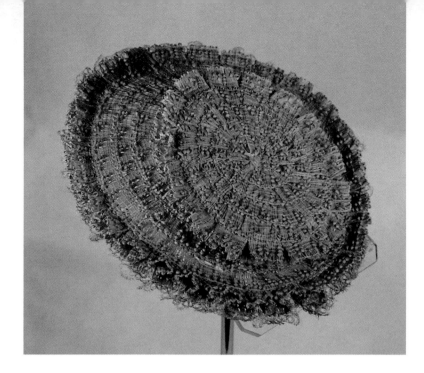

Ca. 1860 elaborately woven open-work, natural straw, trimmed with silk velvet; labeled Geo. Allen, 930 Chestnut St., Philada; Birkenbine Estate.

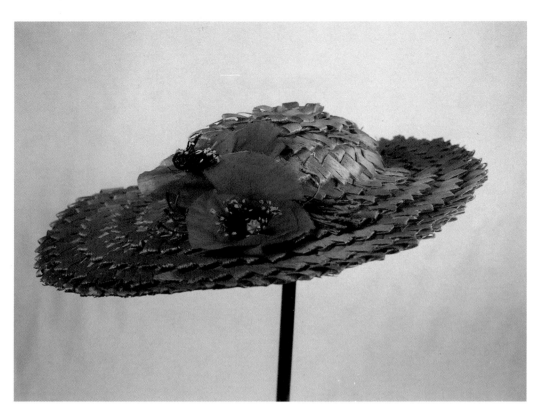

Ca. 1870 loosely woven natural straw, decorated with three small silk poppies, underside of brim is made of tightly woven black straw, lined with silk.

Ca. 1880 plaited natural straw on an intricately constructed wire frame, decorated with silk velvet ribbon, net, flowers, and hand-painted leaves. This hat is very small, 7" in diameter, but weighs a pound!

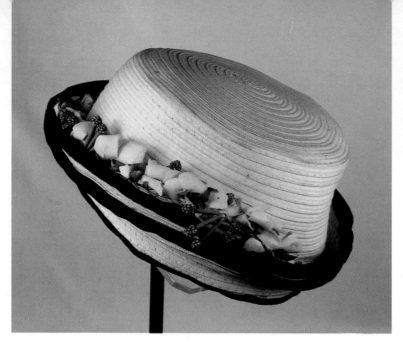

Ca. 1880 fine white woven straw, decorated with black velvet and tiny cloth flowers on one side only, lined in white polished cotton; paper labeled Adele with a picture of an eagle above the name.

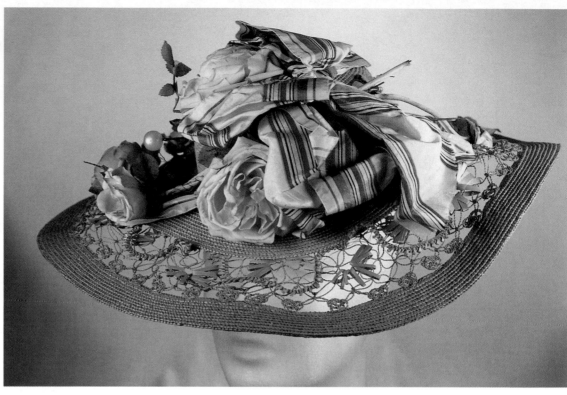

Ca. 1890 natural straw wide-brimmed bonnet, with open-work on brim, cloth roses, colorful striped ribbon on crown and beneath brim; paper labeled, Mrs. F. Herbst, 18 N. 9th St., Reading, PA. *Courtesy of Alison Bartholomew.*

Ca. 1880 finely woven natural straw, shallow crown with a 5" brim, lined with silk chiffon, decorated with a single pale pink silk rose with leaves made of feathers.

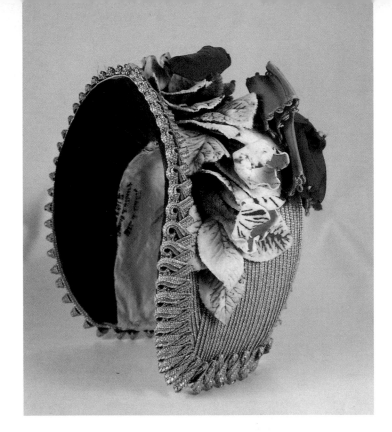

Ca. 1890 natural straw bonnet, trimmed with silk ribbon and velvet hand-painted leaves and flowers with chenille stems, underbrim of burgundy silk velvet; paper labeled for the Columbian Exposition, Chicago, 1892.

In 1890, millinery decorations were called "confections." These confections included fluffy rosettes, pompons, fur, lace, velvet and "most airy flowers in a most indiscriminate fashion." (*The Imperial: A Journal For The Home,* Poughkeepsie, New York, August 14, 1894) In the 1890s, the intriguing thought of the day was that, in fact, "anything may be said to be in the prevailing style."

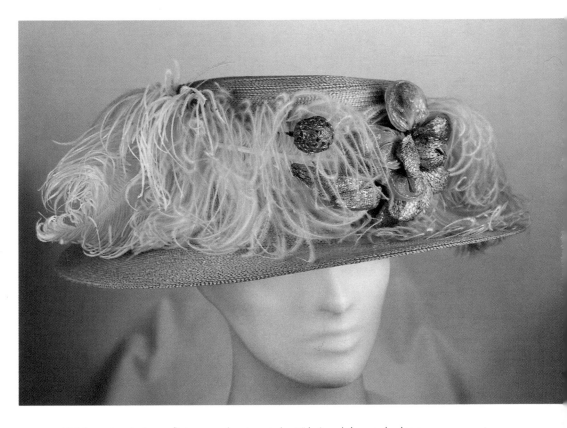

1890s natural straw, flat crown boater style, 3" brim elaborately decorated with an ostrich feather wrap, metallic woven flowers, with silk overlays, and an intricate brass hatpin, cotton lined. *Courtesy of Alison Bartholomew.*

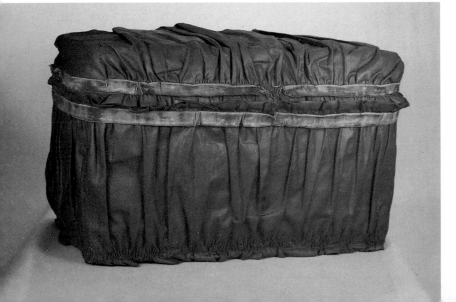

Ca. 1890 basket covered with red polished cotton, this is the original basket for the straw bonnet pictured above, Columbian Exposition.

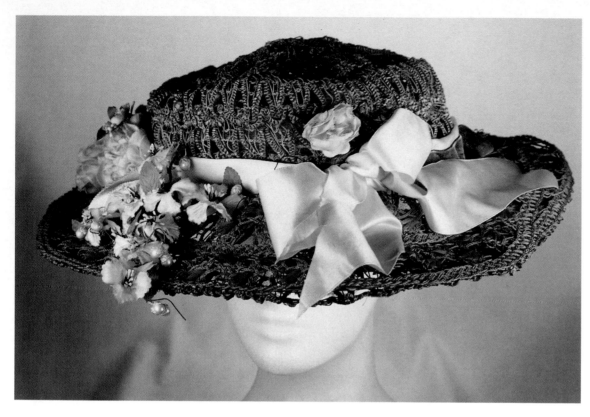

1890s intricately woven, open-work, natural straw bonnet, trimmed with cloth flowers, silk ribbon, and hatpins. *Courtesy of Alison Bartholomew.*

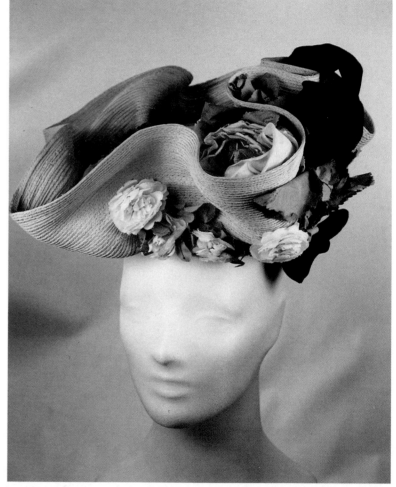

Ca. 1903 natural straw with upswept brim, attached to crown in serpentine waves, cloth roses tucked into folds, trimmed with black velvet bows; labeled Rhind, Brooklyn. *Courtesy of Karen Augusta.*

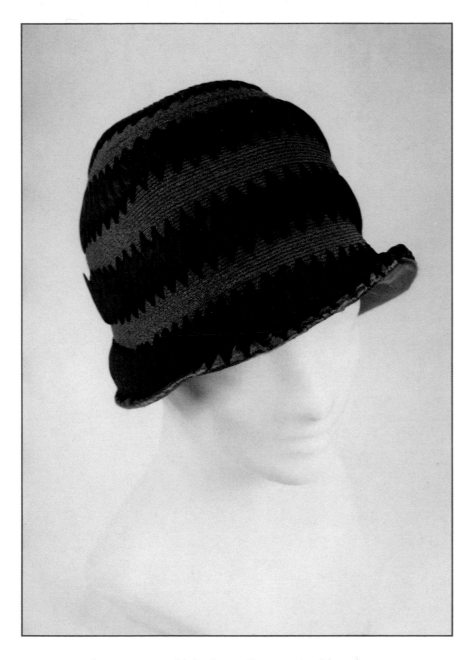

1920s natural straw toque with intricate silk grosgrain ribbon decoration, lined in tan silk; labeled Maxine's Ultra Smart Millinery, 1127
Chestnut Street, Philadelphia.

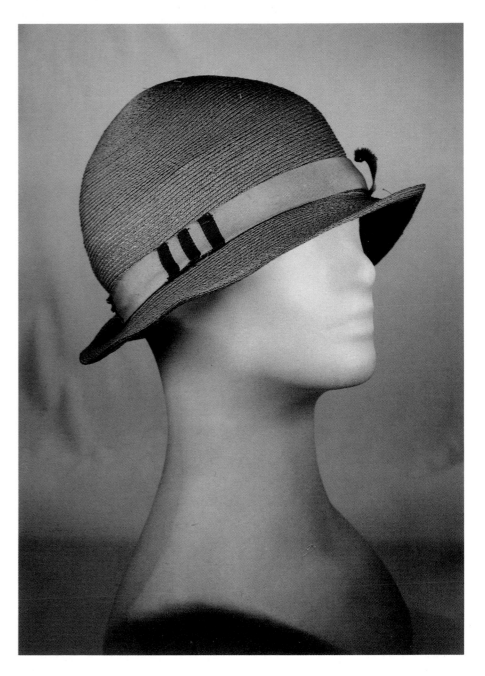

1920s natural straw toque, with tan and brown grosgrain ribbon
band.

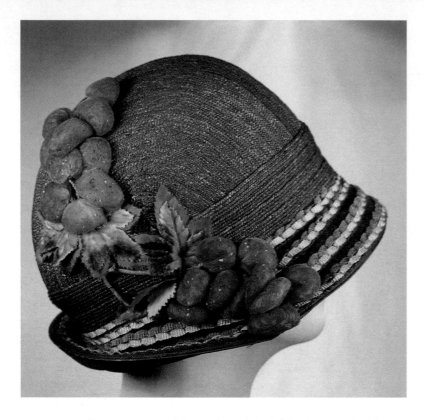

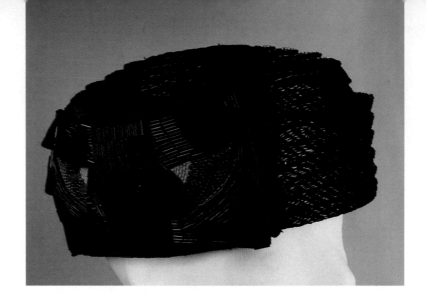

1920s black straw toque, decorated with silk grosgrain ribbon, and glass beads in blue, green, red, yellow, and gray, lined with black polished cotton. A fascinating hat!

1920s natural straw toque, elaborately and colorfully decorated with velvet leaves and plush cotton grapes, covered in sheer orange silk; edged with knitted silk in yellow and orange; silk lined; labeled Darrah & Derr, Fine Millinery, Boyertown, Pa. *Acquired through the generosity of the Women of St. Paul's Episcopal Church, Elkins Park.*

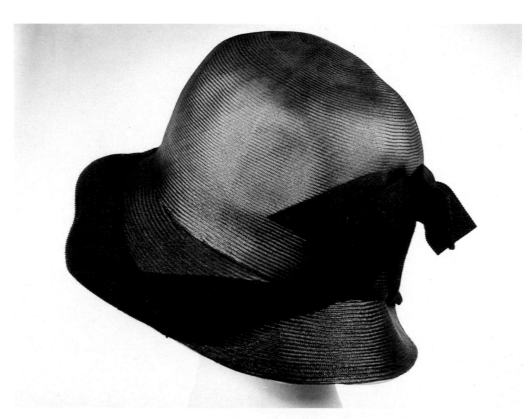

1920s black straw, trimmed with ribbed silk, lined with eggshell silk chiffon; labeled Farguharson & Wheelock, 23 West 57th St., New York, Paris, London.

1930s white synthetic straw, decorated with black and red silk cross-stitches, a red velvet bow, and a single feather; labeled Scharf's, 1633 Chestnut St., Philadelphia.

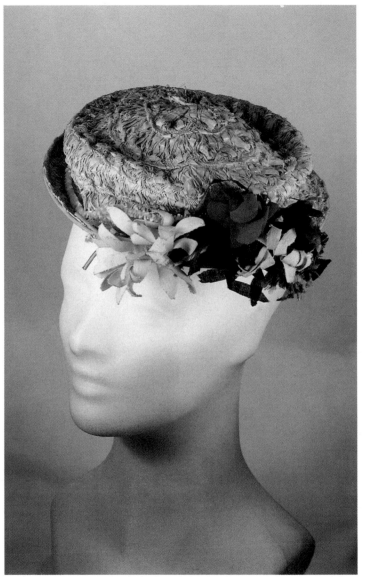

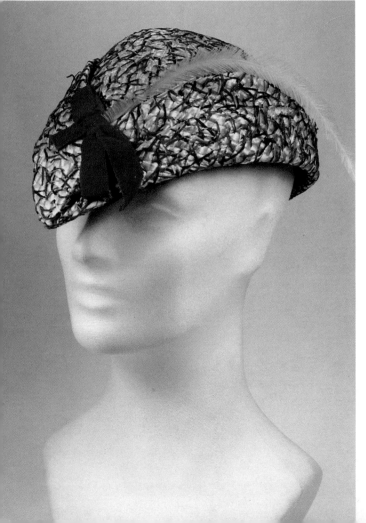

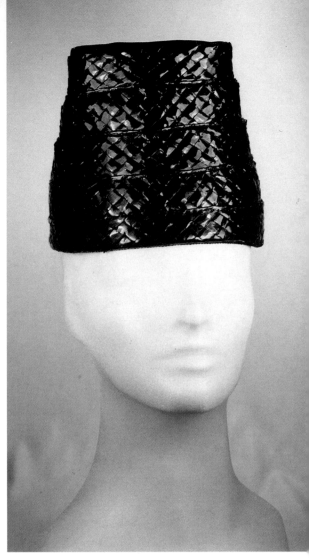

1930s black cellophane straw high-hat, dramatic, brimless styling; labeled New York Creations.

1930s intricately woven straw, trimmed with cloth flowers and leaves.

17

1930s natural straw with green grosgrain ribbon bow and decorative green veil to cover front of rolled brim, tucked up in back with an additional bow under the brim; labeled Coralie, New York.

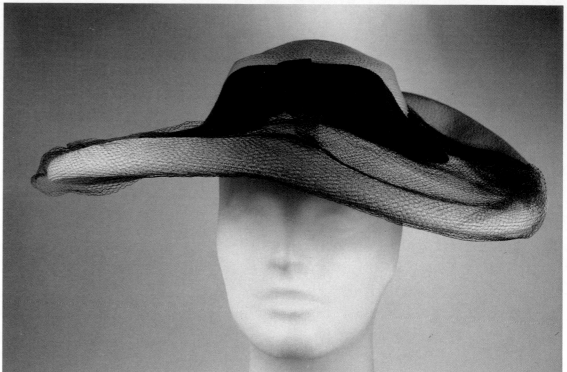

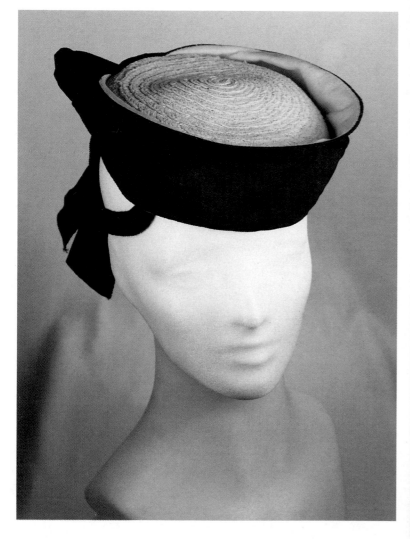

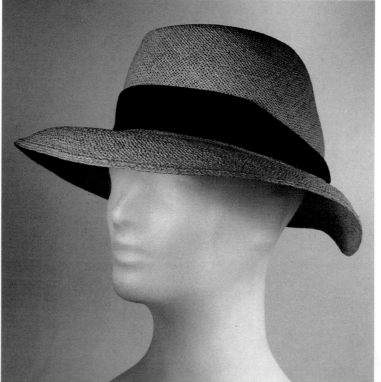

1930s straw "doll hat" with silk grosgrain ribbon around crown and streamers; labeled Paris Maid, New York, Paris.

1940s natural straw with brown grosgrain ribbon band; labeled Stetson Fifth Avenue, Claire Hat Store, Pottstown, Pa.

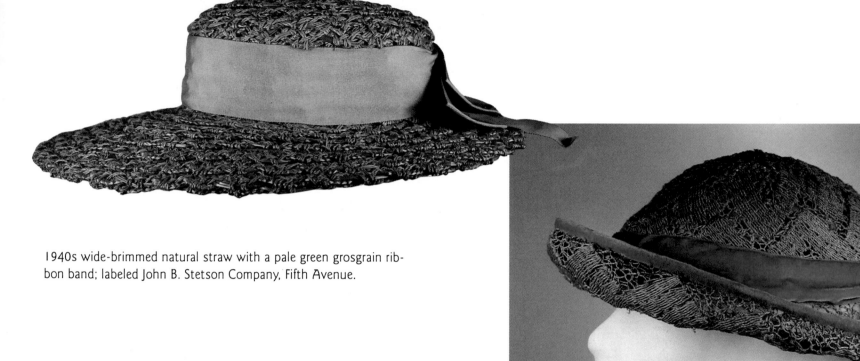

1940s wide-brimmed natural straw with a pale green grosgrain ribbon band; labeled John B. Stetson Company, Fifth Avenue.

1940s woven, open-work natural straw, trimmed with green rayon velvet.

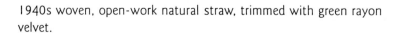

1940s wide-brimmed natural straw with velvet band and streamers; labeled MGM Elizabeth Taylor original. *Gift from Donna Sigler.*

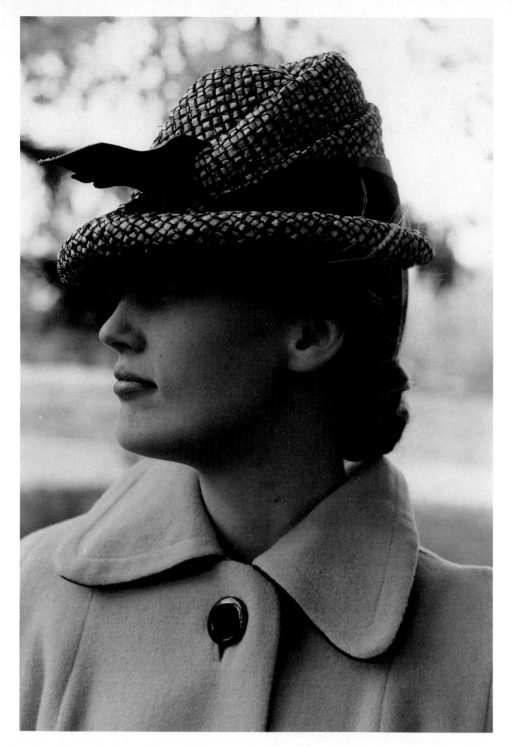

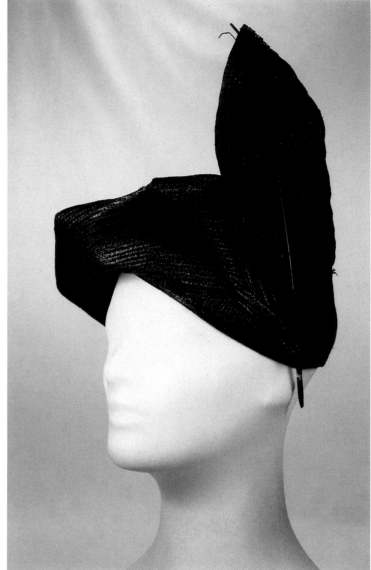

1940s black dyed straw with "feather" decoration, also of straw.

1940s cellophane straw in shades of mauve and gray, with mauve and black grosgrain ribbon; labeled Mr. Milton. *Modeled by Marcie Behanna.*

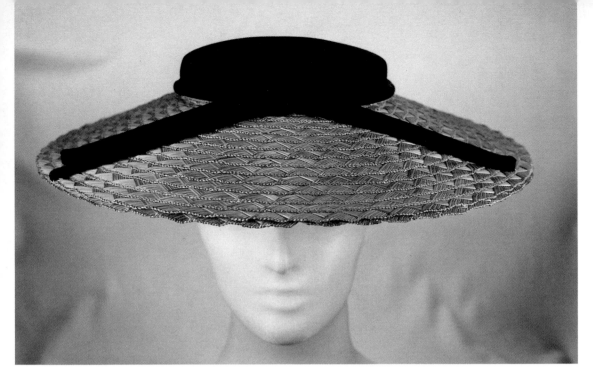

1940s wide-brimmed natural straw with a shallow crown of black velvet and round, black ribbon detailing, extending across the brim. *Courtesy of Lois Fischer.*

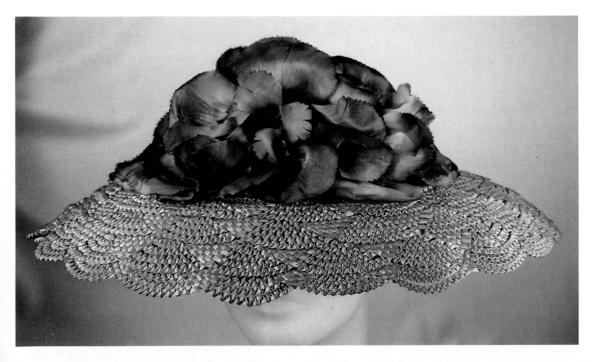

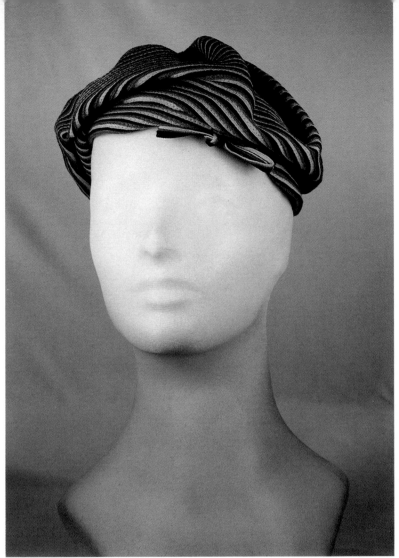

1940s dyed straw in tan, black, and white stripes; labeled Dolly Madison Original, Gimbels, Philadelphia.

1940s wide-brimmed natural straw with scalloped edges, trimmed in mauve and pale green, silk flowers.

Some straw hats that have had lasting popularity are the cartwheel, which has an extra wide stiff brim and low crown; the open-crown which is a halo or toque type hat, having no crown; the picture, which has a large face-framing brim.

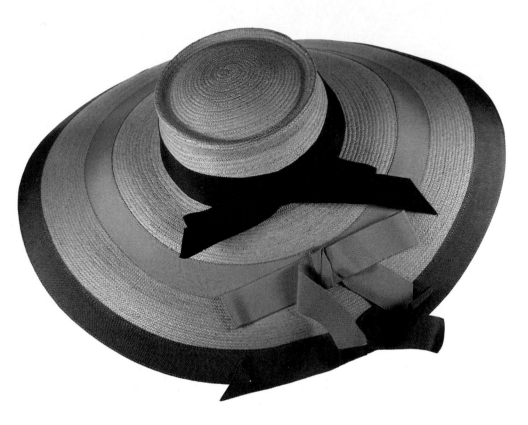

1940s wide-brimmed natural straw trimmed with grosgrain ribbon and bows in shades of green, gold, and brown. A great hat for a garden party!

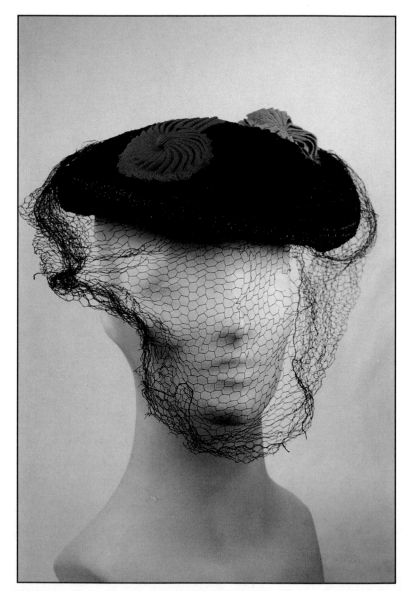

1940s black dyed straw, decorated with intricate grosgrain ribbon "clusters" in black, rose, and gray, veil; labeled New York Creations.

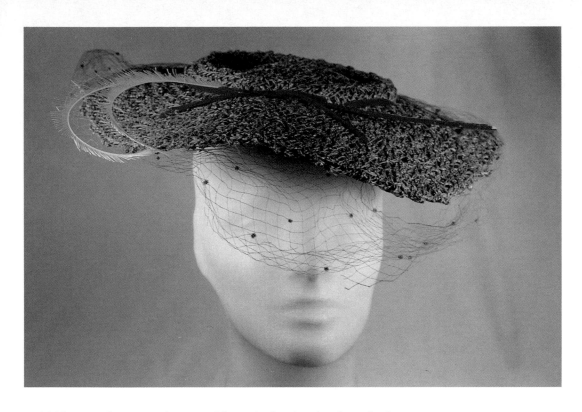

1940s natural open-work straw with a red velvet band and two feathers, beige chenille dotted veil; labeled a Frances Nelkin Offspring.

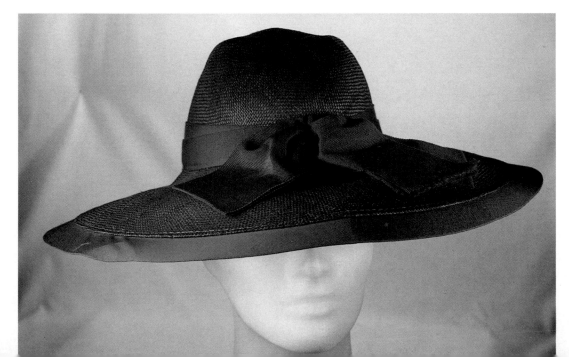

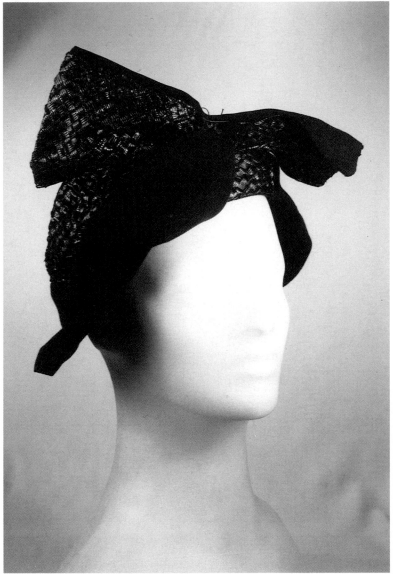

1940s black dyed straw, trimmed with grosgrain silk ribbon; labeled Myrtle Forbes, 5504 Spruce Street, Philadelphia 39, Pa.

1940s brown dyed straw, trimmed with grosgrain ribbon; labeled New York Creations.

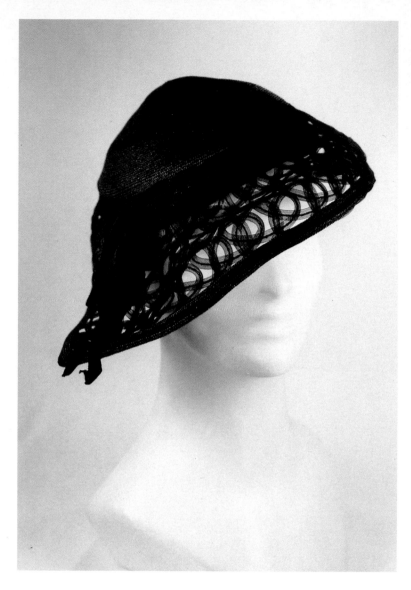

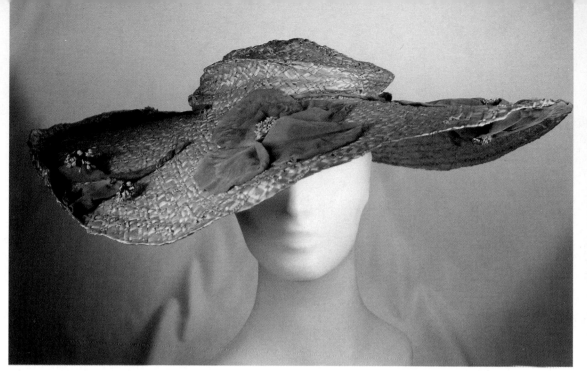

1950s wide-brimmed cellophane straw, trimmed with large velveteen flowers with cloth stems; labeled Hats By Josephine, Claire Hat Shoppe. *Acquired from Ivana Tyler.*

1950s navy straw, open-work brim; labeled Dachettes, Designed by Lilly Daché.

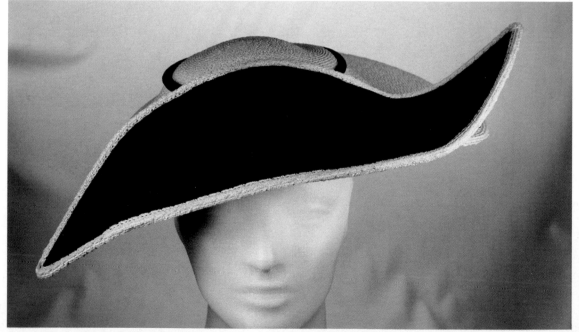

1950s white dyed straw, trimmed in black velvet. Structurally fascinating. *Courtesy of Lois Fischer.*

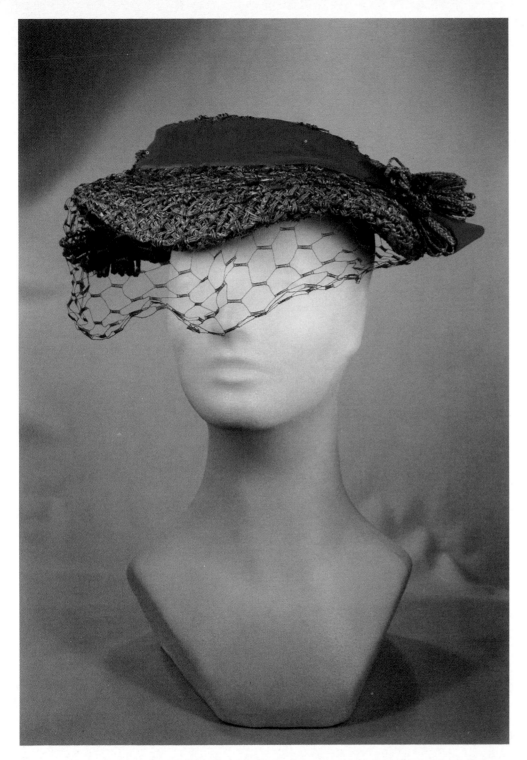

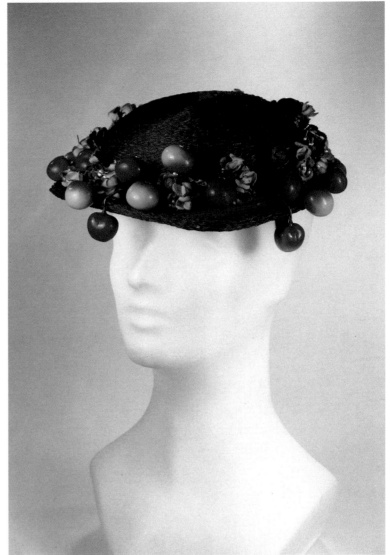

1950s straw, decorated with miniature flowers, beads, and artificial cherries; labeled Dorothy Rose, 1731 Walnut St., Philadelphia, Pa.

1950s natural straw with additional braided straw decorations and orange velveteen ribbon; labeled Hats by Carrols, 174 W. 48th St., N.Y.

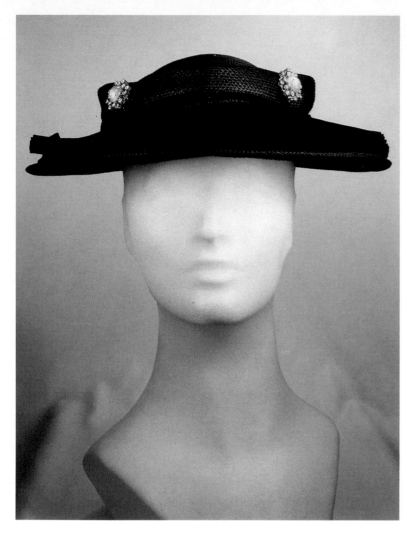

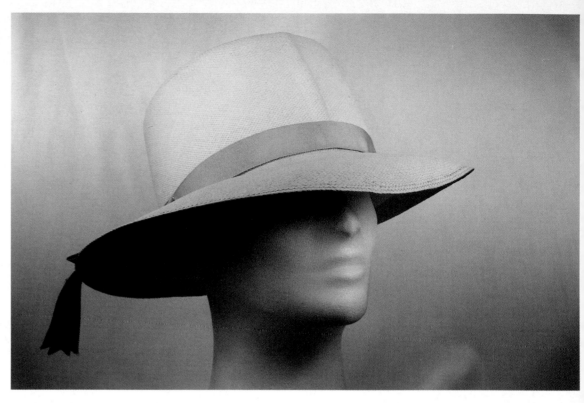

1950s Panama straw fedora with pale green grosgrain band.

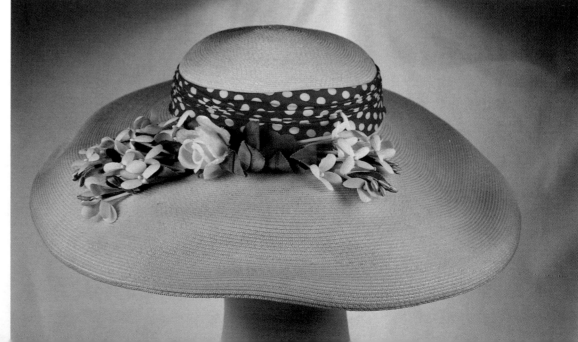

1950s black dyed straw with a pleated silk brim, decorated with two matching rhinestone pins; labeled Fanny and Hilda, 501 Madison Avenue, New York, Leigh Coburn, Philadelphia.

1950s White dyed straw picture hat with a red and white polka-dot band and decorated with white cloth flowers; labeled John B. Stetson Company. *Courtesy of Wear It Again Sam, Manayunk.*

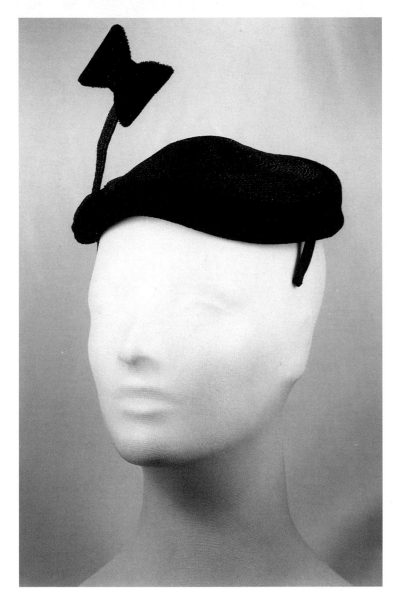

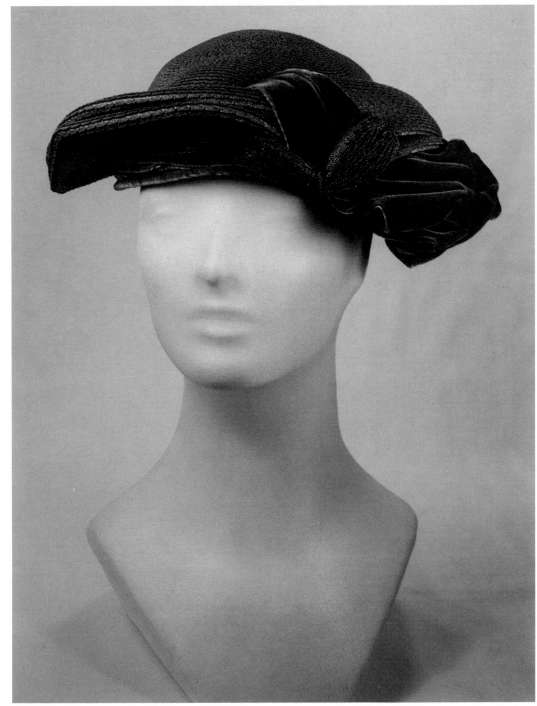

1950s black dyed straw, trimmed with black velvet and a "stand-up" bow.

1950s blue dyed straw, trimmed with blue silk velvet ribbon and glass beads. Great structure!

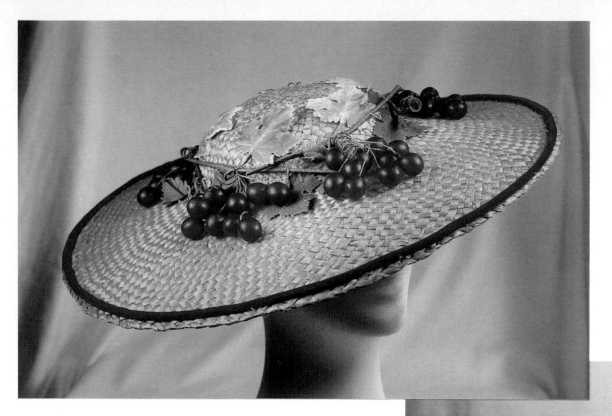

1950s natural straw picture hat, trimmed with bunches of burgundy grapes and green leaves, with a single round velvet ribbon edging the large brim; labeled Custom Made Laddie Northridge, 16 W. 57th St., New York. *Courtesy of the Drexel Historic Costume Collection, Nesbitt College of Design Arts, Drexel University.*

1950s natural straw with Oriental lines, tied with a scarf of black silk chiffon.

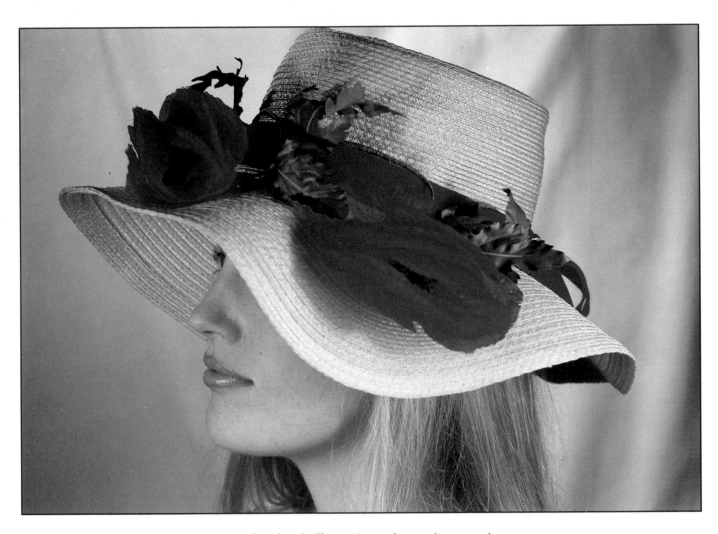

1950s straw, decorated with red silk poppies and green leaves, red velvet ribbon band with a bow in back; labeled Mr. Kurt Original, Miss Bea Mack. *Modeled by Marcie Behanna.*

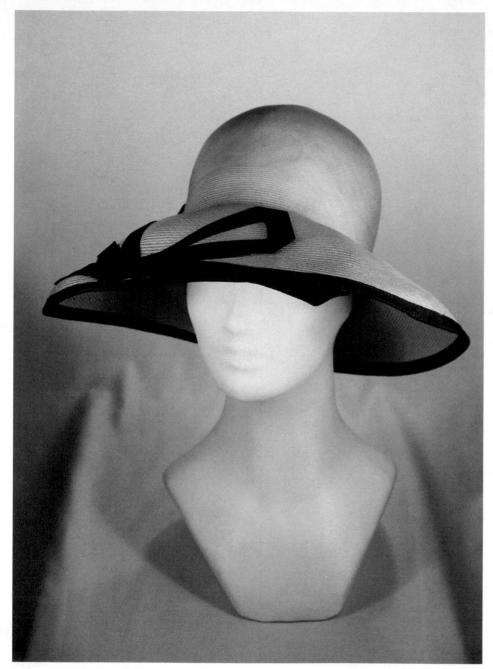

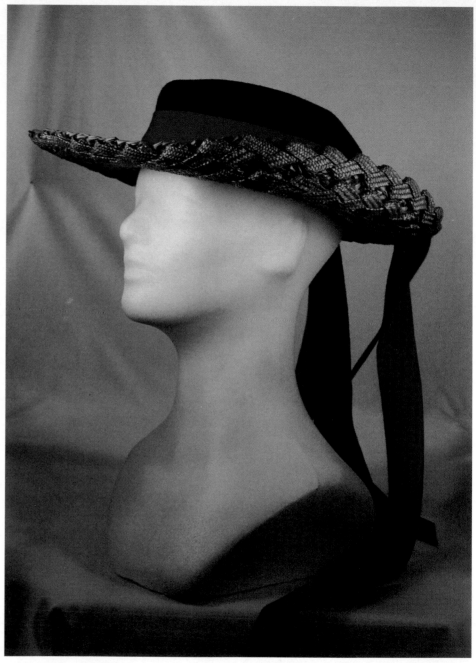

1960s natural straw, trimmed with black grosgrain ribbon; labeled Frank's Girl, Designed by Frank Olive, New York.

1950s wide-brimmed natural woven straw, with a black felt crown and grosgrain ribbon streamers; labeled Leslie James.

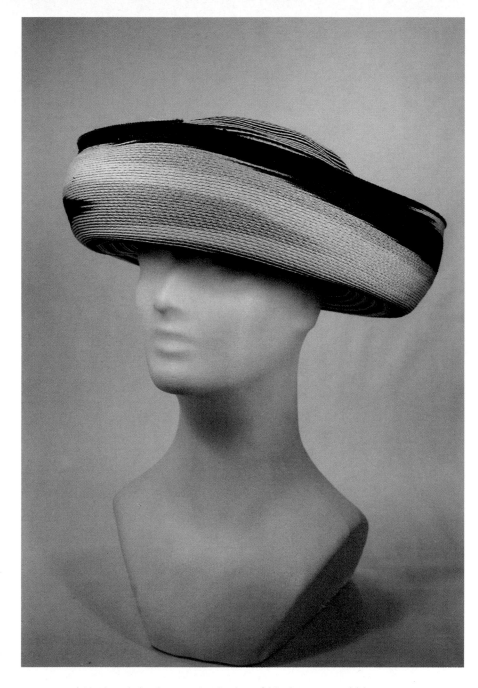

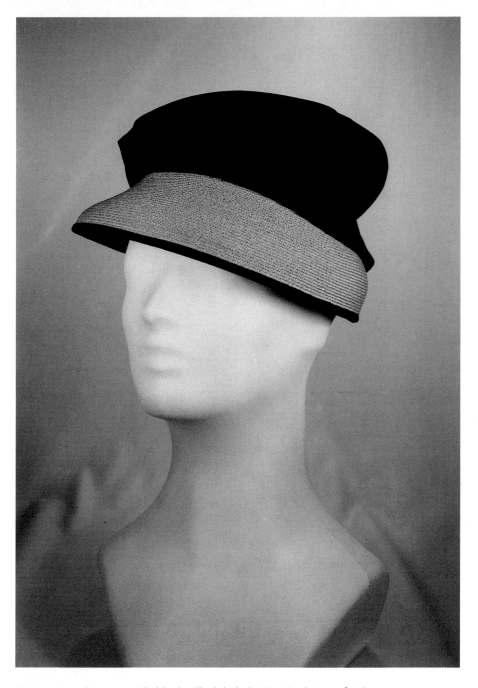

1960s multi-colored dyed straw in shades of black, gray, and blue; labeled Hess Brothers, Allentown, Pa.

1960s natural straw with black silk; labeled Miss Frederics of John Frederics, New York.

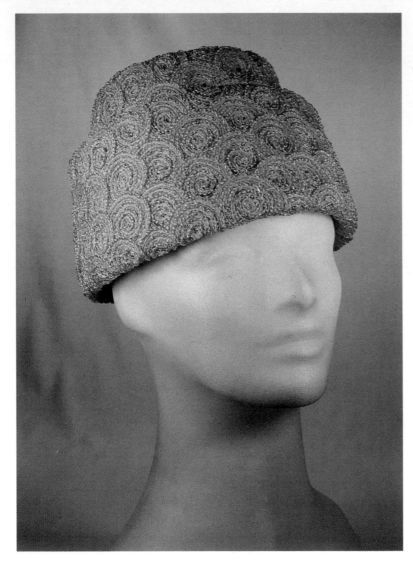

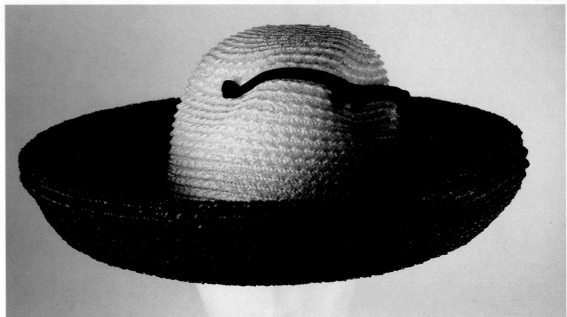

1960s straw with a white crown and navy turned-up brim; labeled Mr. Kurt Original, Miss Bea Mack.

1960s straw, made of many small intricate circles stitched on a net base; labeled Saks Fifth Avenue.

1960s avocado green dyed straw, with a velvet ribbon band and turned-up brim; labeled Mr. Kurt Original.

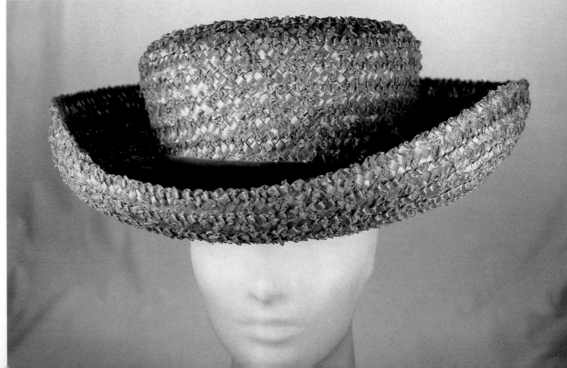

🐇 Felt 🐇

Fur felt hats from 1850 to 1890 have survived in surprisingly large numbers. Many of these hats have very wide brims, four to eight inches from the crown, and can be twenty-four inches in diameter or even wider. These hats are usually found in excellent condition, rarely showing the moth and rodent damage characteristic of many of the later felts. Often the wide-brimmed fur felt hats are without decoration. This may be because trim was removed and reused on another or later hat. Some of the plain fur felt hats I have acquired, show signs of having had trim or decoration at one time. Loose threads, or remnants of silk, sequins, or jet beads are visible around the crown. Since many of the hats were worn for mourning, this would also explain why so many are plain, or decorated only with black ribbon or ruching (trim that is pleated and stitched so that it ruffles on both sides).

When I first started collecting hats, I assumed that most fur felt hats were beaver. Unfamiliar with the felt making process I expected the hats to be as thick as beaver pelts. Many of the hats are actually made of beaver, as the underfur of the aquatic mammal is apparently notched and well adapted for felt making, since the fibers interlock easily. During the 19th century "beaver" became a generic term for any kind of fur felt hat.

Eventually, restrictions were placed on beaver hunting and the use of fur from the coypu, the rabbit, and the hare began to take over. *Putnam's Home Cyclopedia Hand Book of Useful Arts* (New York, 1852) tells us that a good beaver hat required about two and a half ounces of a mixture which included eight parts of rabbit fur, three parts of Saxony wool and one part of llama, vicuña, or red wool. The formula for a good "beaver" hat includes no beaver!

No adhesives are used in felt making. Some felts are hard and smooth; others are soft and napped. Velour is soft and velvety. Originally felt was made of all wool yarns, but recently it has included other fibers.

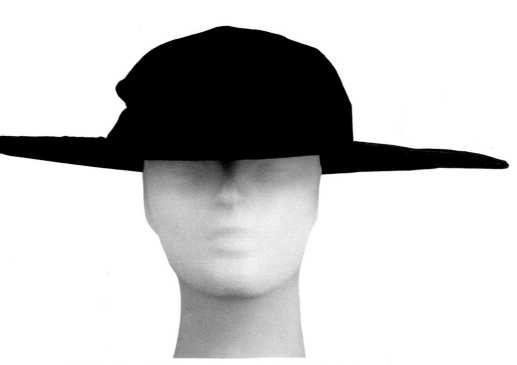

1880s black fur felt wide-brimmed hat; underside of brim is silk velvet. The silk lined hat is 18" in diameter.

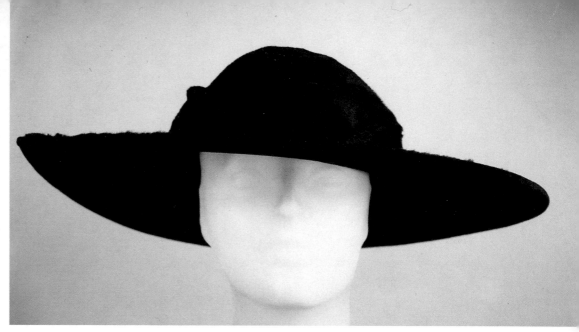

1880s black wide-brimmed "beaver" hat, silk lined, exceptionally high quality.

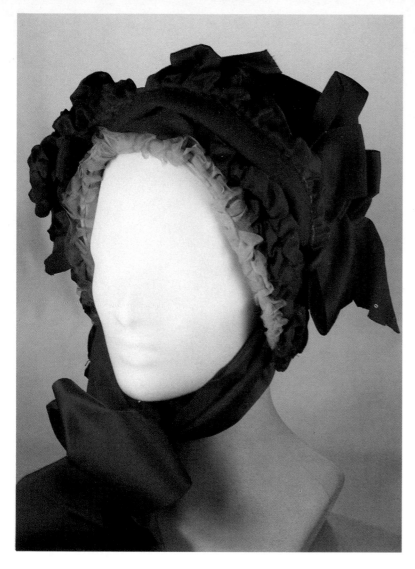

1880s red felt bonnet, trimmed with red silk ribbon, wide red silk ribbon ties, padded and lined in eggshell silk, tulle edging. By tradition, these bonnets were made of "worn out" cloaks, because the red felt was so highly prized.

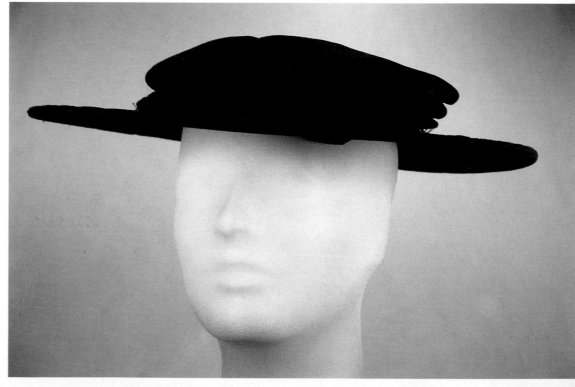

1880s beaver "flat hat," lined with black silk.

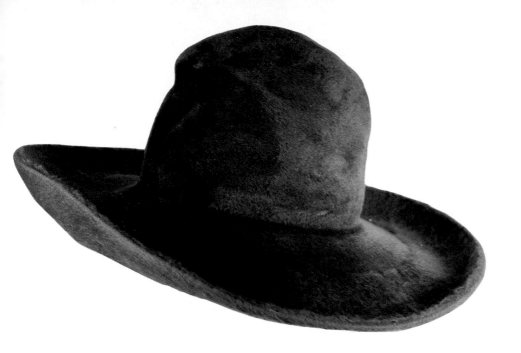

1880s avocado green fur felt broad brimmed hat, high crown, shaved fur felt on brim, showing two levels, labeled in paper, for ordering, suggests French origin.

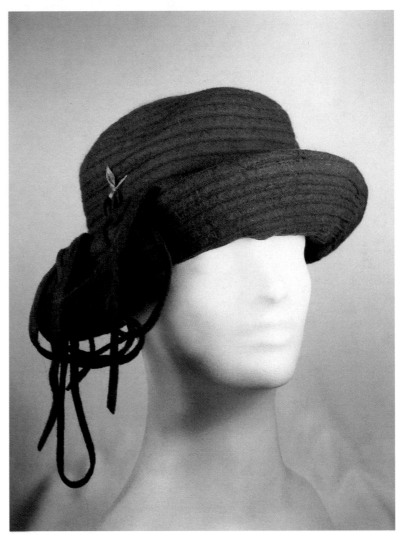

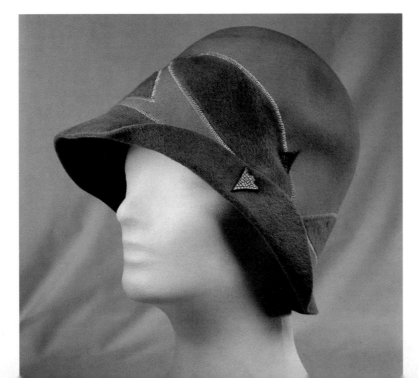

Ca. 1900 chestnut brown fur felt, with polished cotton lining. One of my personal favorites. This hat is stitched together using a technique generally reserved for straw.

1920s toque, tan felt and velour, with copper "arrow" hat pin; labeled Seaman and Townsend, 45 West 51st Street, New York. *Courtesy of the Drexel Historic Costume Collection, Nesbitt College of Design Arts, Drexel University.*

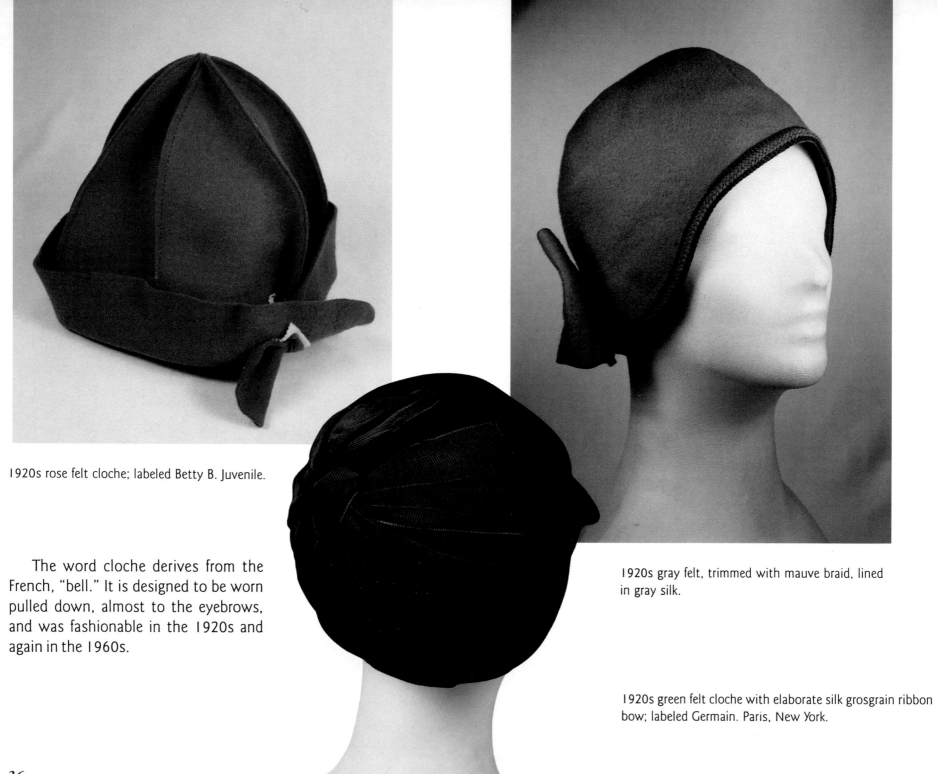

1920s rose felt cloche; labeled Betty B. Juvenile.

The word cloche derives from the French, "bell." It is designed to be worn pulled down, almost to the eyebrows, and was fashionable in the 1920s and again in the 1960s.

1920s gray felt, trimmed with mauve braid, lined in gray silk.

1920s green felt cloche with elaborate silk grosgrain ribbon bow; labeled Germain. Paris, New York.

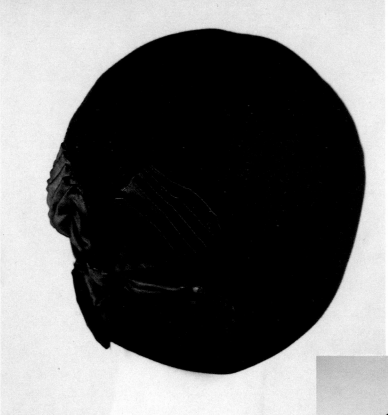

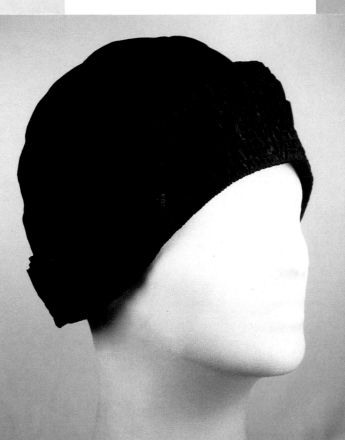

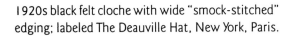

1920s black felt toque with criss-cross felt brim and elaborately tucked silk bow in back; labeled copy of Original Agnes, Paris.

1920s black felt cloche with wide "smock-stitched" edging; labeled The Deauville Hat, New York, Paris.

1920s black felt toque.

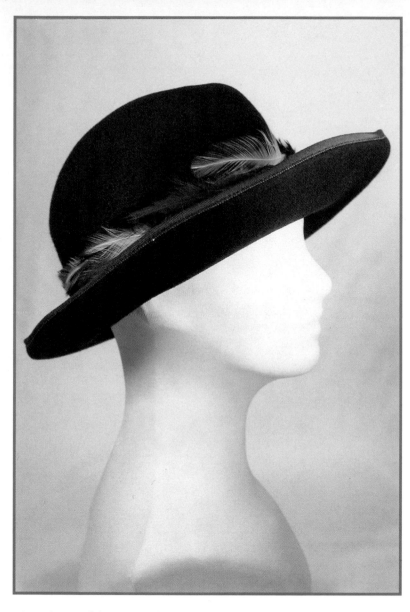

1930s brown felt, trimmed with tan and brown feathers; stamped inside crown Astar, 100% wool.

The fedora hat was popularized for men after Victorian Sardou's play *Fedora* was produced in 1882. It was not long before it was being designed in felt for women also, and it has remained popular ever since.

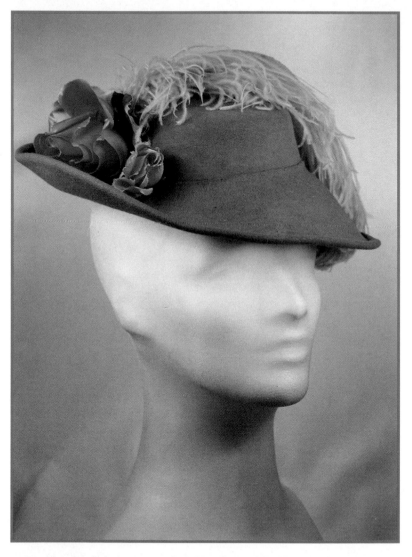

1930s blue felt fedora, trimmed with pink sweetheart roses, blue silk bow, and a blush pink ostrich plume; labeled Mme. de la Barre, 10 W. 55th St., N.Y., Paris. Owned by Countess Mara de Bninska, who was also the milliner. *Courtesy of Karen Augusta.*

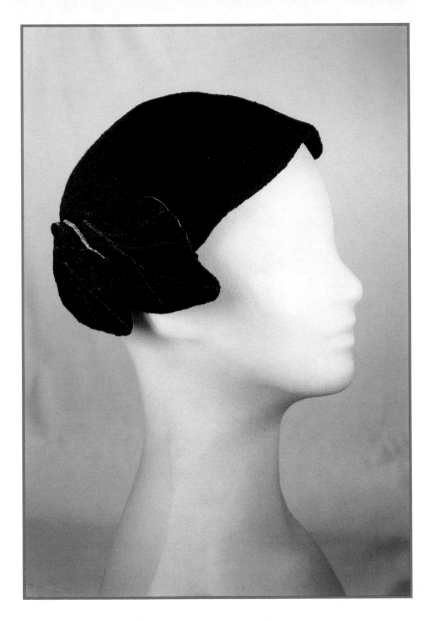

1930s green felt detailed with four cloth padded ivy leaves; labeled DeLacy, 425 Park Ave. Near 55th St., New York.

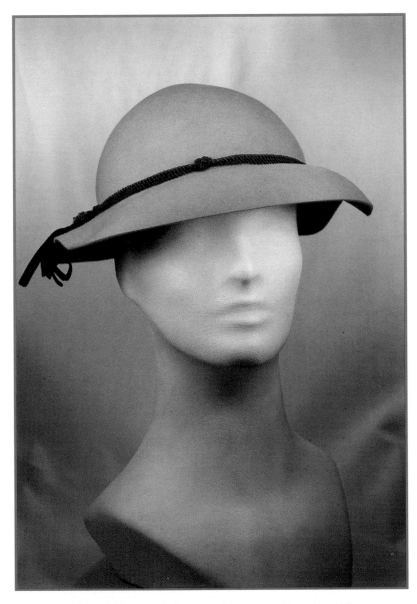

1930s tan felt with a rounded crown, brown cord band, and brown kid decoration; labeled Dobbs, Fifth Avenue, New York. This is a rare example of a woman's hat made by Dobbs. Filene's, Style D66, Color Sandy Beige, Price 7.

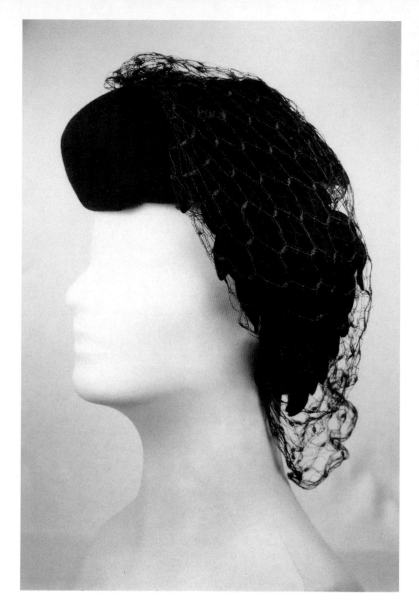

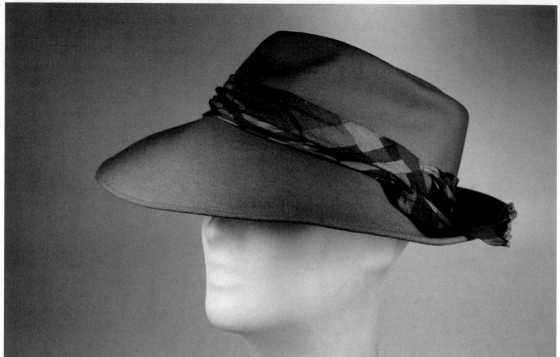

1930s tan felt with a madras plaid band in shades of green, yellow and blue; stamped inside crown Berkshire, Made in U.S.A., Mohn.

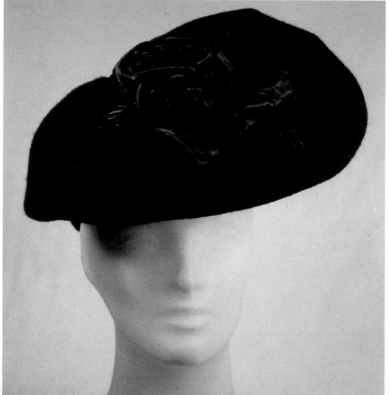

1930s brown felt with felt "feather" decoration and large mesh veil in back; labeled E. W. Edwards & Son, Rochester, Syracuse, Buffalo.

1930s brown felt with large brown velveteen roses and an open crown; labeled Beltone hats, New York.

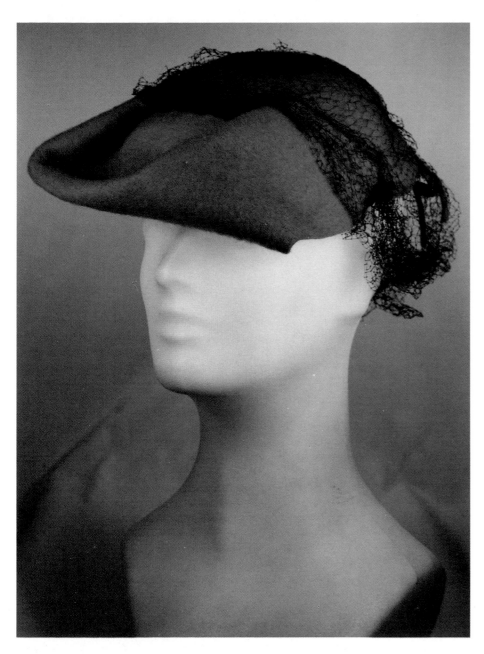

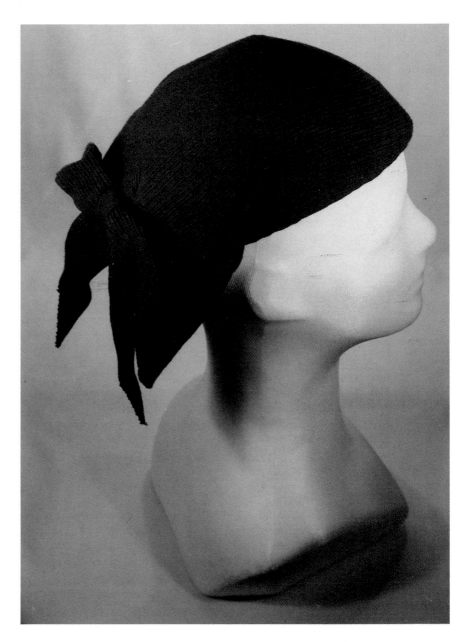

1930s mustard-colored fur felt with brown veil and a bow in back.

1930s blue ribbed felt, bow in back, lined in black silk chiffon; labeled LeBonnet, Chestnut Hill, Phila.

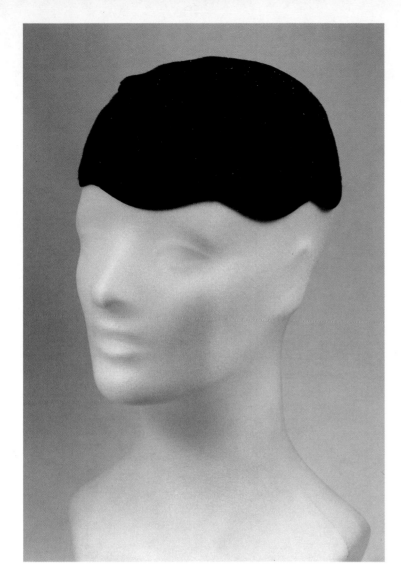

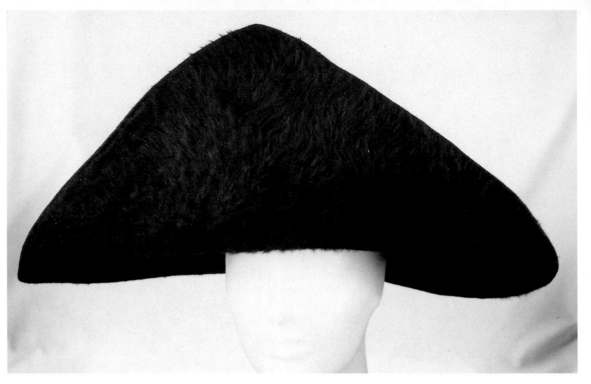

1930s black fur felt, brim shows tricorne effect.

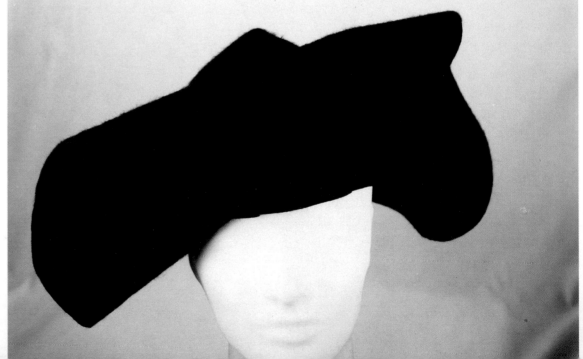

1930s black velour skull cap; labeled Hattie Carnegie.

1930s black fur felt, made up of eight separate pieces.

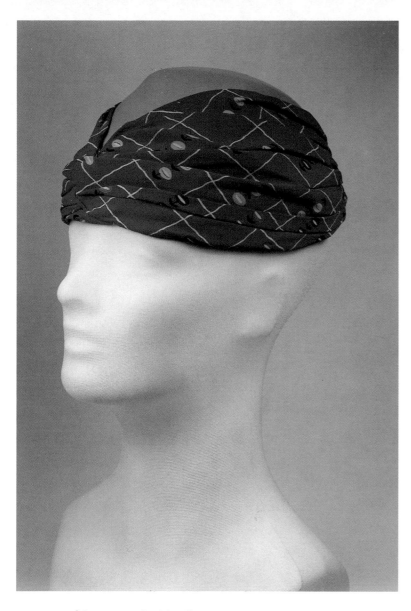

1930s tan felt, wrapped with silk rayon geometric print, "scottie" type.

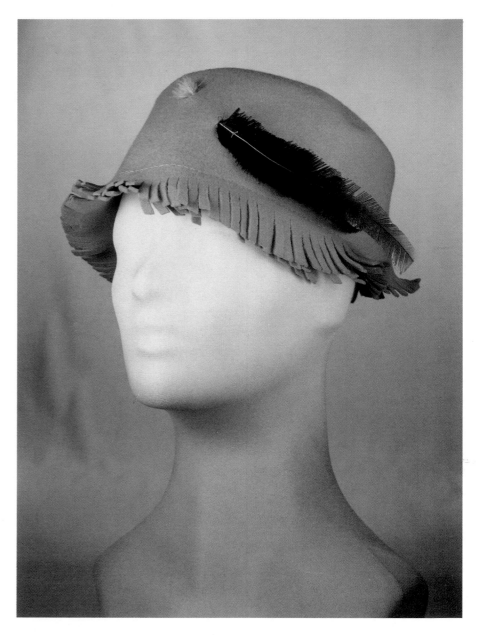

1930s pink felt with a fringed edge and trimmed with two feathers; stamped inside crown Glenover, Henry Pollak, Inc.

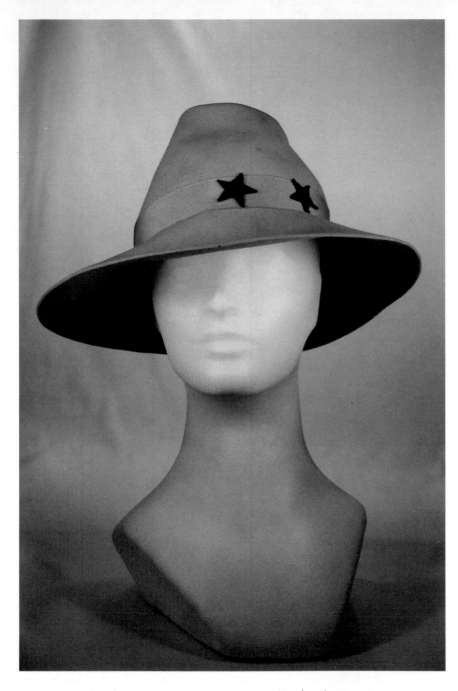

It is somewhat difficult to distinguish among several types of felt hats for women which were popular during the 1940s and 1950s. The swagger is an informal sports hat with a medium sized brim, turned down in front. The snap-brim has a brim that may be worn at several different angles. The slouch, or Garbo hat, has a flexible brim which may be turned down in front. The ever popular fedora has a medium sized brim, high crown, and a crease from front to back.

Stetson

John B. Stetson, the most well known manufacturer of hats in the world, so well known that his name is virtually synonymous with the western or cowboy hat, made women's hats too—lots of them. The women's hats were shipped from the factory in Philadelphia to various locations, large department stores, and small millinery shops. Many of the Stetson women's hats are labeled John B. Stetson, Fifth Avenue or John B. Stetson, 1224 Chestnut Street. Women who shopped regularly at the Stetson store on Chestnut Street in Philadelphia have told me that most of the hats in the store were for men, and that the women's hats were in the "back of the store."

The original Stetson Factory has been demolished, but the business still exists and is currently owned by Resistol Hats, a Texas firm. Although the company continues to offer a selection of Stetsons for men, it only occasionally produces western hats for women, and has not produced any of the earlier fashion hats, such as those pictured here.

1930s yellow felt fedora, with a grosgrain ribbon band and two navy "stars"; labeled John B. Stetson, Fifth Avenue.

Trends in Millinery

The cloche and the mushroom brim define the 1920s. Picture hats became increasingly popular as women ventured more often into the afternoon sun. Cloches were embroidered with metallic and silk threads. Although hat bodies were commonly made of felt, often overlays of cut velvet or elaborate beading on net were used. Horsehair, mixed with silk, was used to create a light flexible millinery texture for the enduring garden parties. Sports clothing for women increasingly demanded appropriate millinery.

The 1930s is represented by a manly bunch of soft felts for daytime wear. This comfort and durability was juxtaposed against some structurally diverse, if not surrealistic, cocktail and evening hats. Felt was the material of choice, and geometric lines, rather than soft curves, dominated design.

The 1940s styles are eclectic. Interrupted by the war years, material conservation, and women in the work force as never before, it is not surprising that the hats of this period were extremely functional. Until the war ended, fewer women went out socially, and because of this the more frivolous styles were not popular until the late 1940s. Seasonal shopping sprees for appropriate millinery again became derigueur.

The millinery business reached its heyday in the 1950s. Post war prosperity for the middle class, and the return to routine and formality in dress, fed a slavish conformity to morning, noon, and night millinery.

A stylish first lady heralded in 1960s millinery. Wearing a large pillbox and fashionable, simple lines in clothing and accessories, Jackie Kennedy captured the attention of the nation. Too quickly, with our young President's assassination, did our attention as a nation turn away from a family's fashionable lifestyle to the very serious concerns of the Civil Rights Movement and protesting the Vietnam War. Hair became a universal symbol of rebellion. In the face of sweeping social change, the hat diminished in importance.

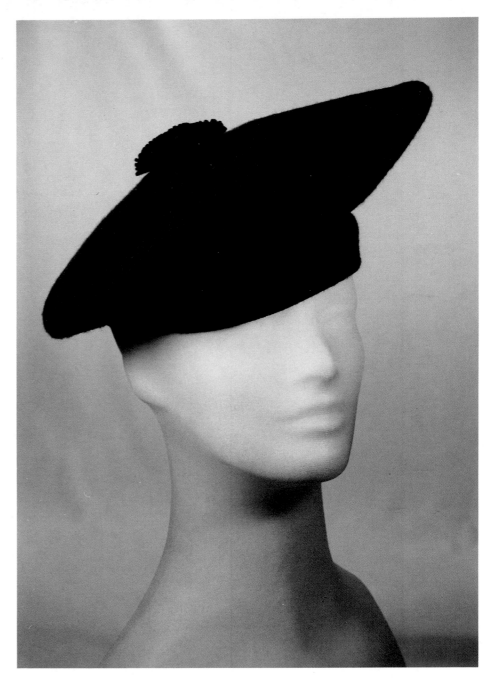

1930s navy felt, modified tam-o-shanter.

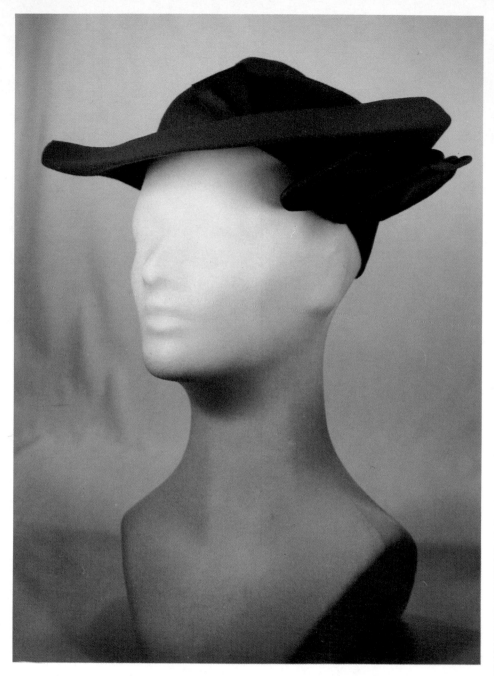

1930s burgundy velour with silk satin ribbon "pulled through" the brim; stamped inside crown, Merrimac Ritz.

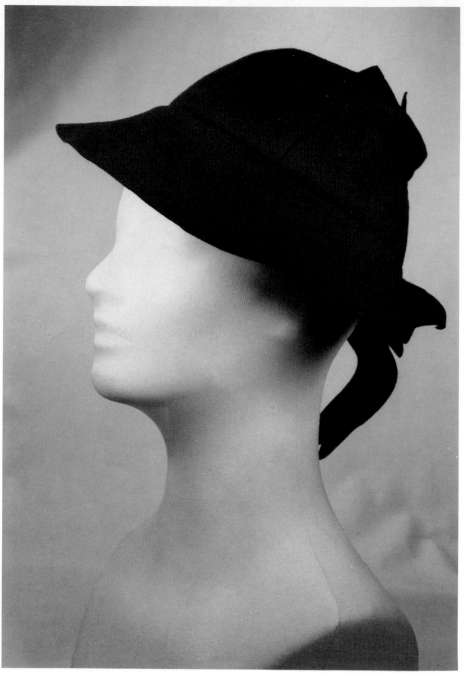

1930s rust brown velour, with a self-tie back.

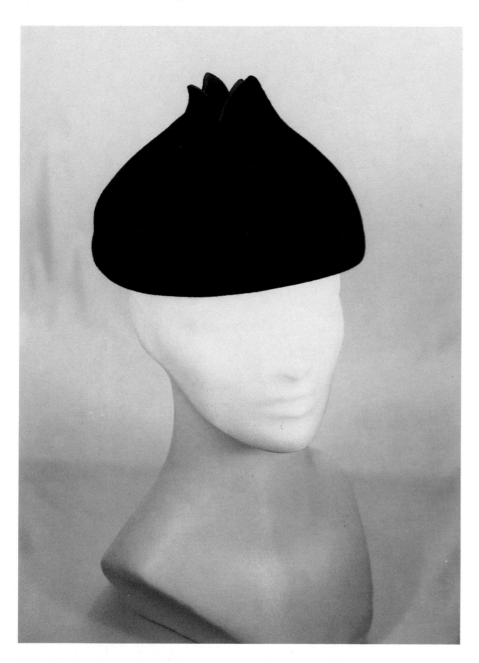

1940s black velour, with an open crown detailed with red felt; labeled original design by Madcaps, New York.

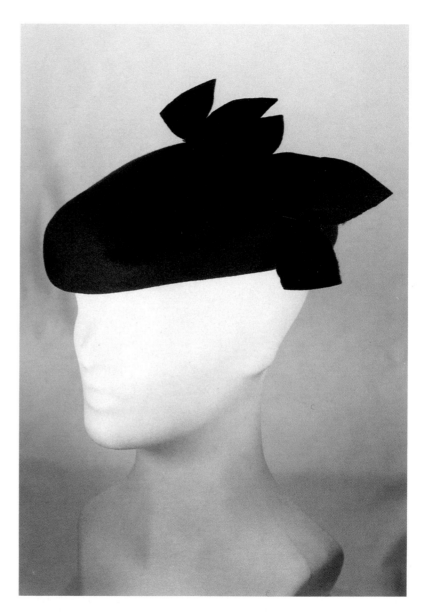

1940s brown felt with "stand-up" bow decorations; labeled New York creations.

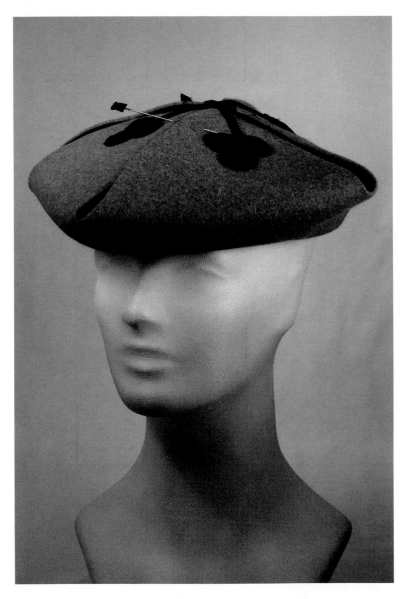

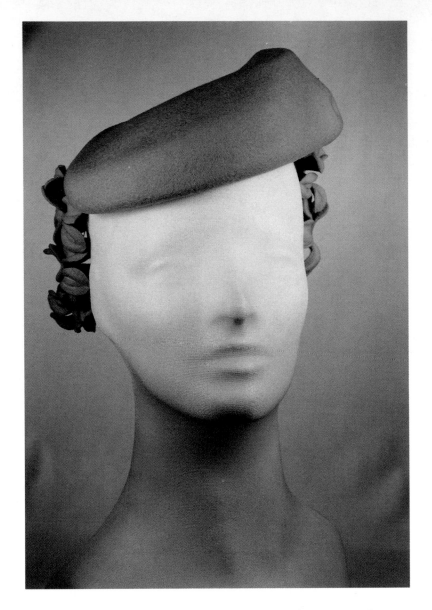

1940s chartreuse felt with felt flowers; stamped inside crown Merrim Hat Corp.

1940s tan felt tricorne, lined with brown satin; labeled Leslie James, Hess Brothers, Allentown, Pa.

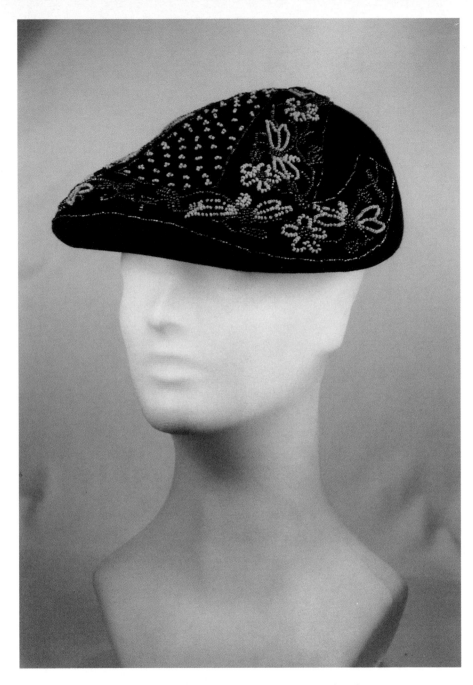

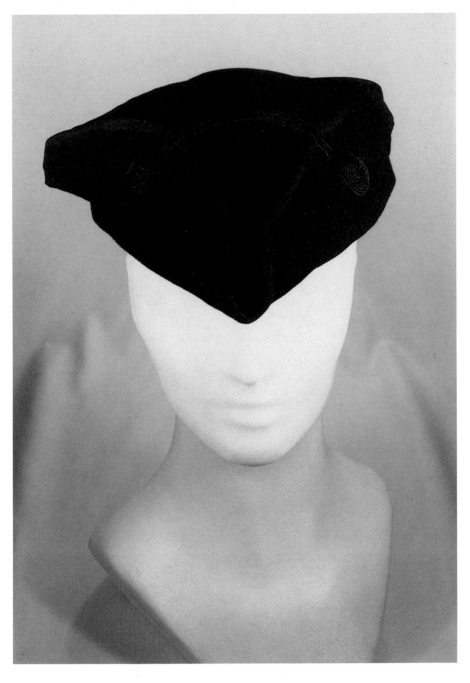

1940s black felt "sports inspired" hat, decorated with glass beads in shades of blue, pink, and gray.

1940s black fur felt, trimmed in cord and grosgrain ribbon, tricorne shape; labeled Madelon, 55 Brompton Rd, S.W.I.

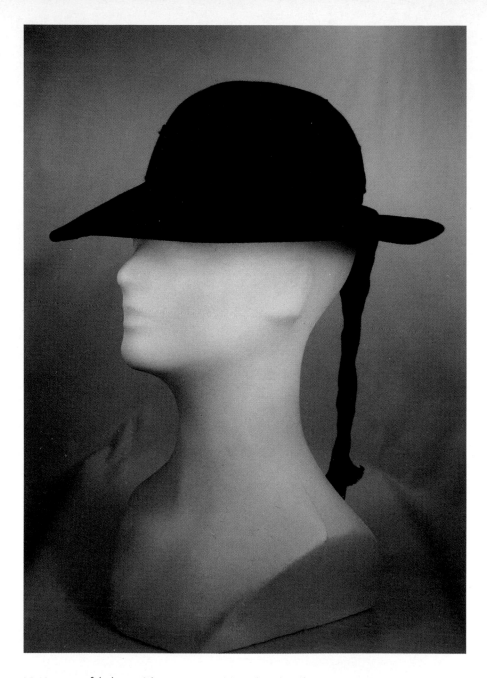

Hollywood Style

Hollywood has always influenced fashion. What the stars wore in 1930s films represented the glamour missing in everyday life. The at-home catalogs, such as Sears, 1935, showed "autographed fashion" hats for Dorothy Wilson, Alice White, Ann Southern, and Adrienne Ames. In the 1940s the Cinderella Hat Company made hats commemorating the child stars Elizabeth Taylor, Judy Garland, and Margaret O'Brien. Hollywood designers, such as Gilbert Adrian, designed the most extravagant, exciting styles for the stars, and women copied those styles in their daily lives, especially in millinery trends.

Traditions

Wearing hats in church goes back to the early tradition that women's hair was so distracting to men, so seductive, even blasphemous, that it should be covered. Hats were considered to be decorative and fashionable, but certainly better than a woman's uncovered head.

The tradition died slowly. The more traditional religious groups continued the custom. In some churches, particularly African-American churches, many women continue wearing hats to express a sense of formality, an appropriateness of dress. As Betty Pearson of *Hatitudes* said, "In my community hats never went out of style. Many women still believe that you're not dressed unless you have a hat on your head."

1940s navy felt hat with grosgrain ribbon band and streamers; labeled MGM Filmstar, Judy Garland, Hat by Cinderella, New York, Chicago. These hats are very special and not easy to find.

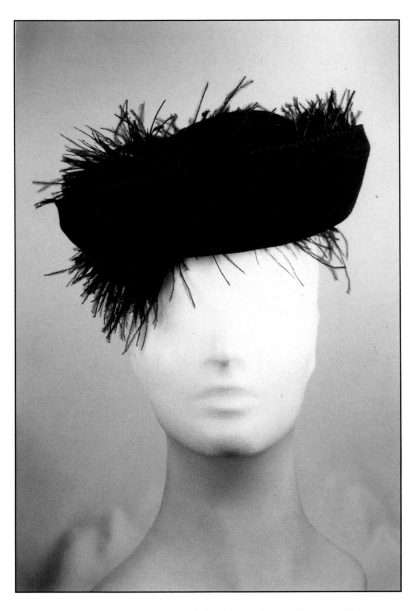

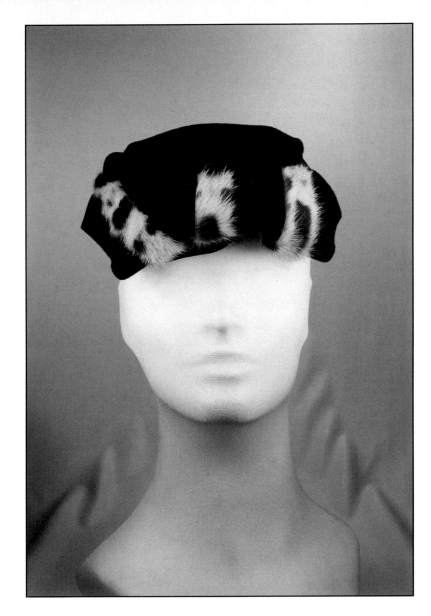

1940s brown velour, trimmed with strips of leopard fur.

1940s navy felt trimmed in ostrich feathers; labeled Glenover, Henry Pollak, Inc., New York.

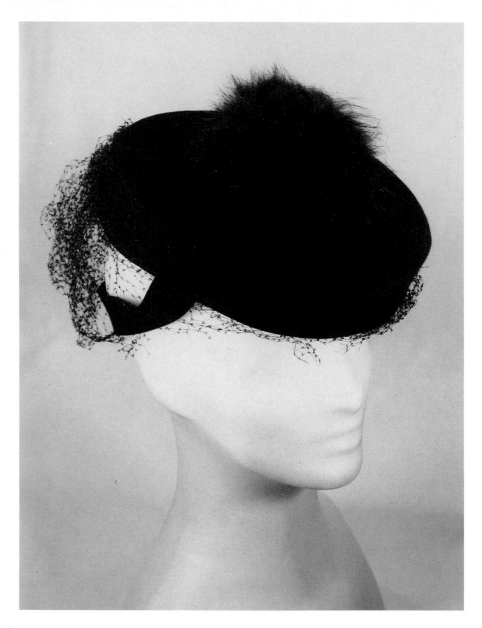

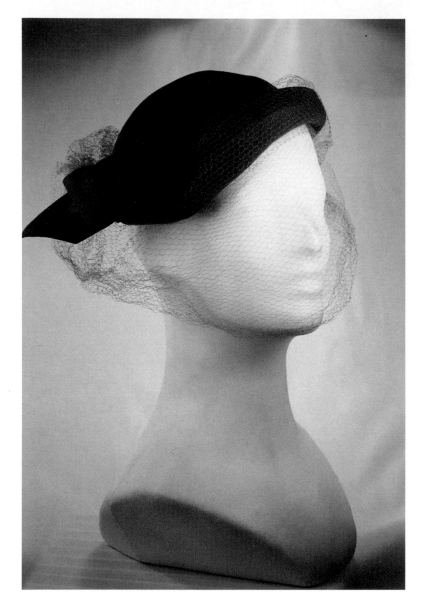

1940s black felt with a fur ponpom on top, veil; labeled The Heinz Store, Scranton, Pa.

1940s green felt with veil; labeled Jean Allen, Styled by Sage.

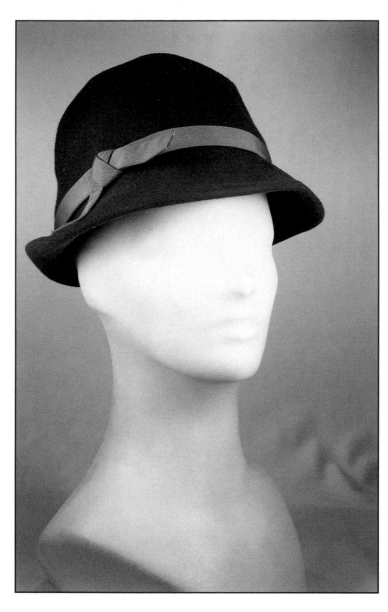

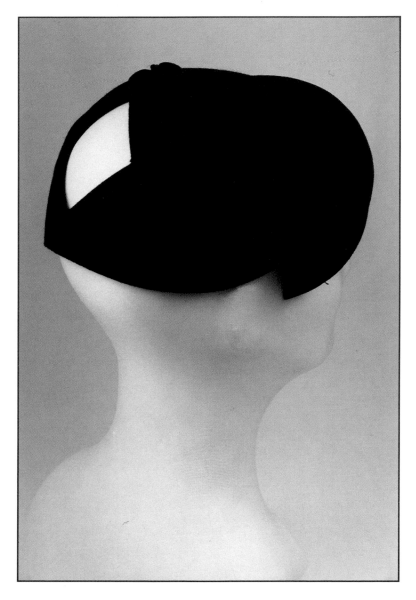

1940s tan felt fedora with grosgrain ribbon band; labeled Lilly Daché, Paris, New York, Tribout Shop, John Wanamaker.

1940s black felt with stand up ridges at sides, and tight skull cap with an open diamond in back; labeled New York Creations.

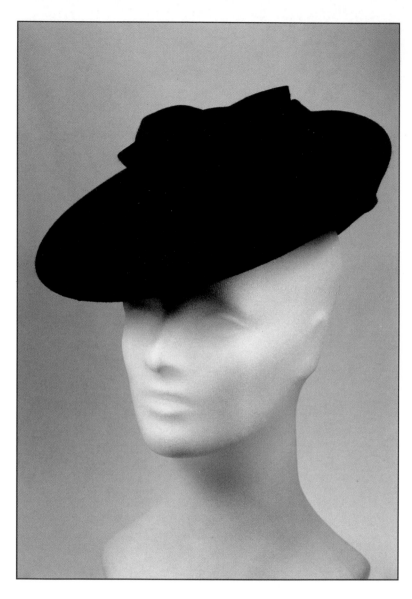

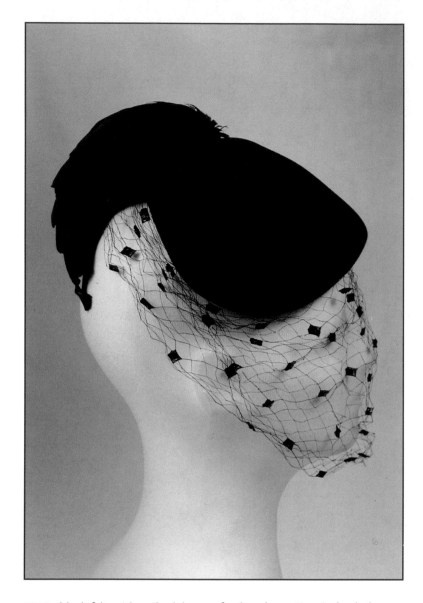

1940s navy felt with "stitched" designs. Interesting geometric shape.

1940s black felt with veil, elaborate feather decoration in back; labeled Fred Phipps, New Haven, Conn.

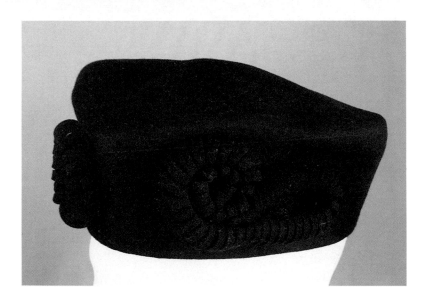

1940s black felt with intricate designs of twisted felt strips on sides.

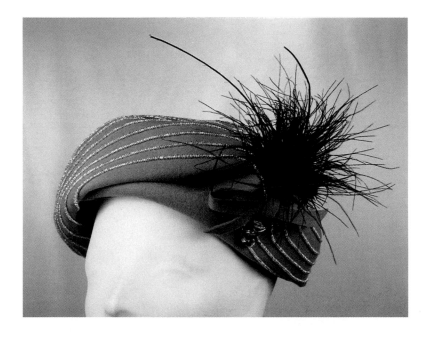

1940s tan felt trimmed with silver metallic cord and one feather.

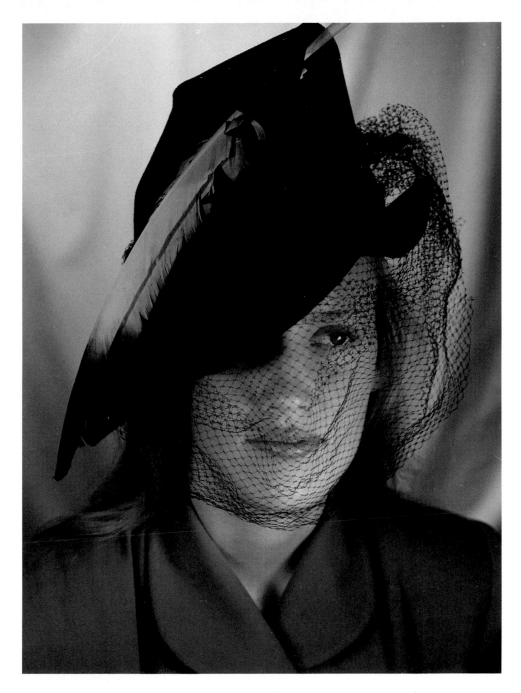

1940s black fur felt with feather and veil; labeled Norman Durand Original. *Modeled by Marcie Behanna.*

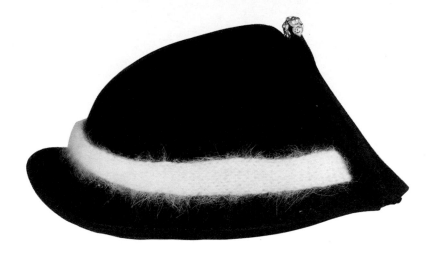

1940s dark brown velour, trimmed with angora knit trim, rhinestone "ball" on back; labeled John B. Stetson Company, Fifth Avenue.

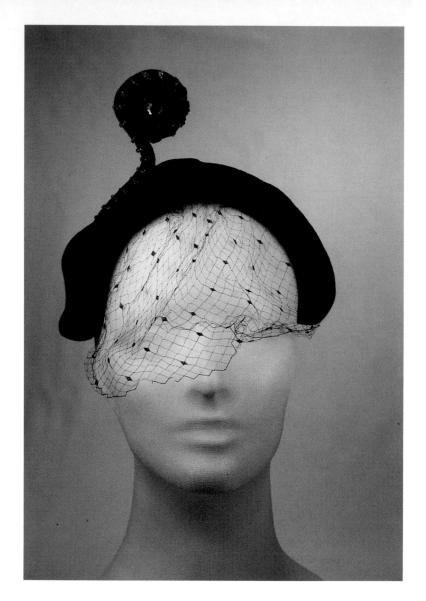

1940s black velour with stand up, beaded decoration, and chenille dotted veil; labeled Brandt, New York, Paris, H. Leh & Co., Allentown.

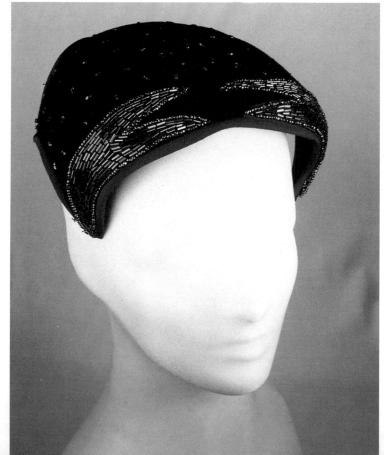

1940s "clip type" velour, trimmed with copper bugle beads.

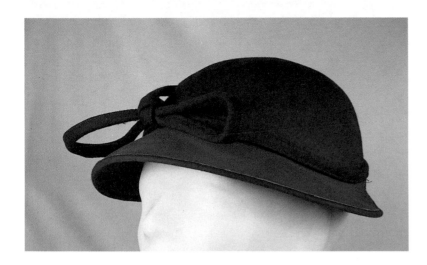

1950s green felt with tan suede brim and felt bow.

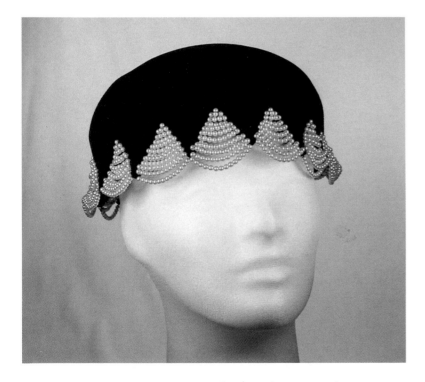

1950s black velour trimmed with artificial pearls in triangular rows; labeled The Blum Store, Philadelphia, stamped Aurole, Made In France.

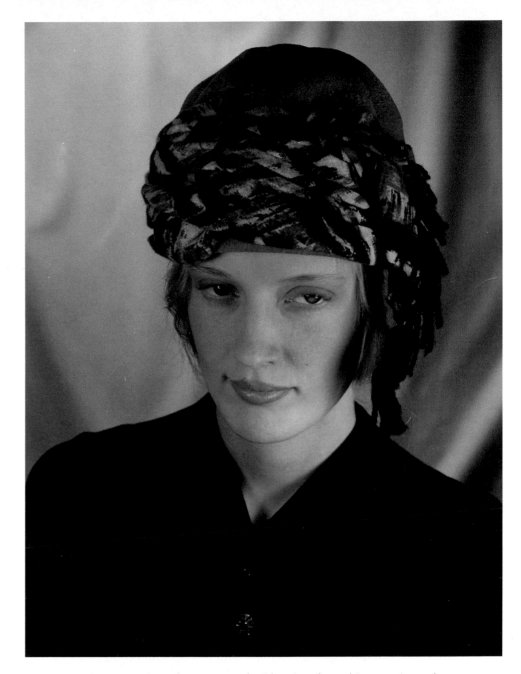

1950s turquoise velour, wrapped with printed wool jersey trimmed with black wool; labeled Lilly Daché, Paris, New York, Young Modes. *Modeled by Marcie Behanna.*

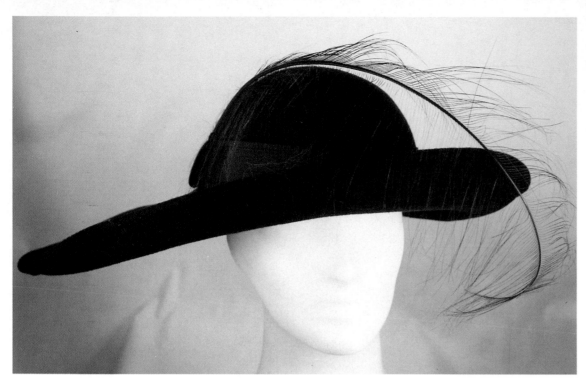

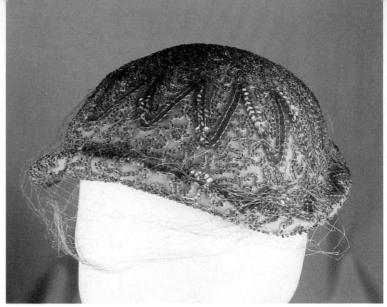

1950s pink felt covered all-over with silver glass beads, and salmon colored sequins, veil; labeled Stetson, 1224 Chestnut Street, Philadelphia.

1950s deep purple felt asymmetrical brim with grosgrain ribbon band and a single feather; labeled Mr. John Classic, New York, Paris.

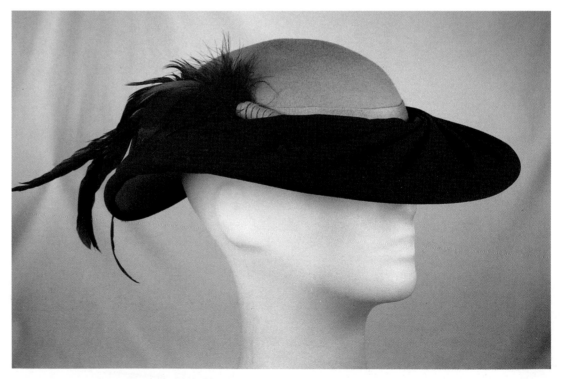

1950s pink Doeskin felt with a burgundy velour gathered brim; trimmed with a few feathers; labeled Designed By Sylvia, New York, St. Louis.

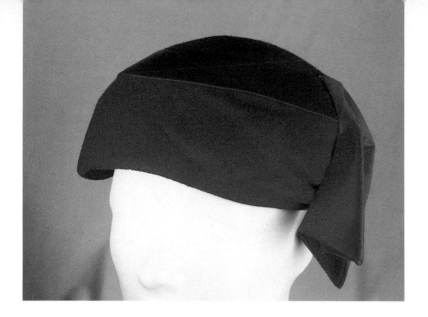

1950s red felt, trimmed with satin; labeled Glamour Felts, Terry Sales Corp., N.Y.

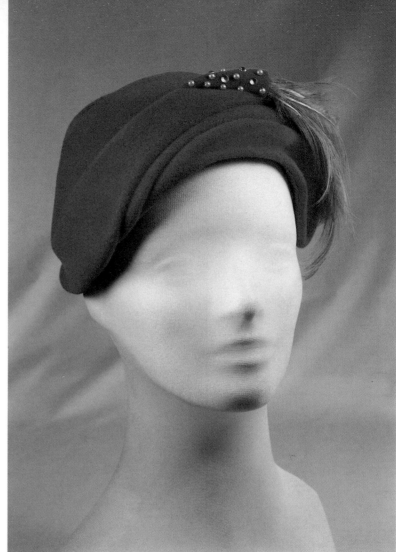

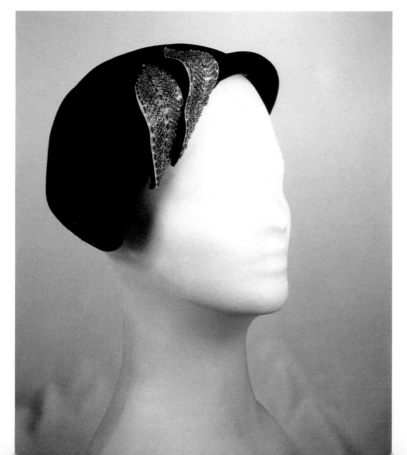

1950s salmon colored felt decorated with pearls and rhinestones and a single feather; labeled Hess Brothers, Allentown. *Courtesy of the Drexel Historic Costume Collection, Nesbitt College of Design Arts, Drexel University.*

1950s black felt with silver silk "feathers" decorated with glass beads; labeled Stetson, 1224 Chestnut Street, Philadelphia.

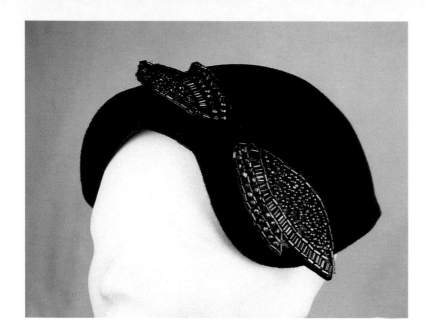

1950s brown fur felt trimmed with "leaves" of copper bugle beads, and a felt bow.

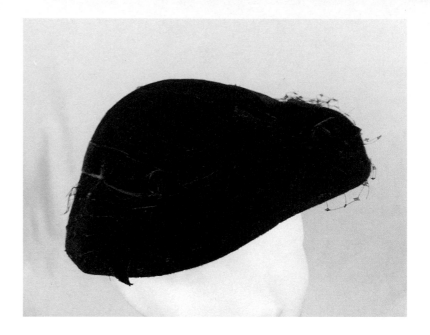

1950s navy velour hat, trimmed with velvet bows and veiling; labeled Reproduction of Albouy, 49 Rue Du Colisée Elysée 91-23, Paris.

1950s tan velour, purchased at Lit Brothers, grosgrain band and back ribbon. *Courtesy of Katherine Stauffer.*

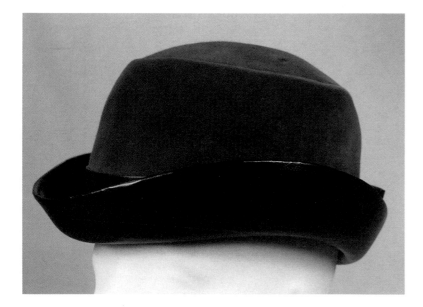

1950s brown velour "riding hat" with a black leather brim; labeled Lilly Daché, Tribout Shop, John Wanamaker.

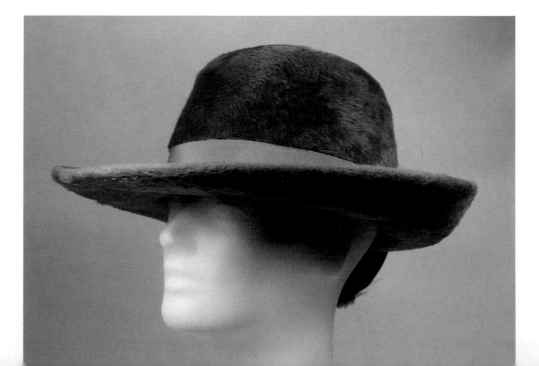

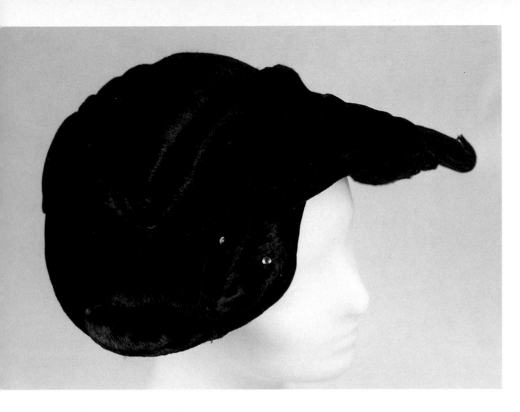

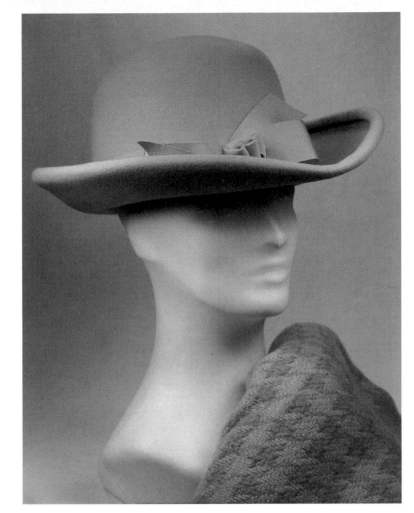

1950s black and blue fur felt, trimmed with velvet and rhinestones. Fascinating shape.

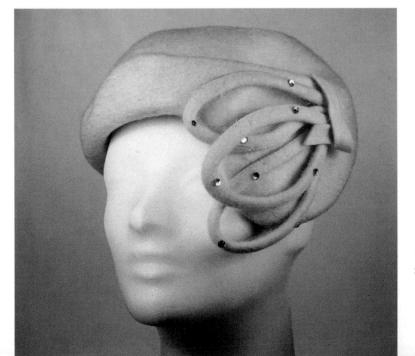

1950s pale turquoise velour with a grosgrain ribbon band to match. Designed by Danny Weil for Katherine Stauffer, to match a suit, fabric pictured. "Danny Weil could design anything." *Courtesy of Katherine Stauffer*.

1950s oyster white velour, trimmed with rhinestones; stamped inside crown Merrimac Hat Corp. Great detailing.

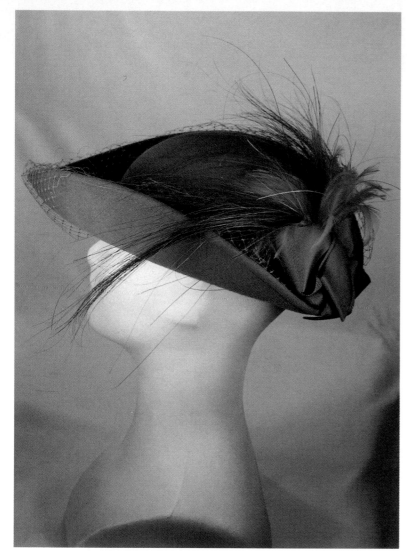

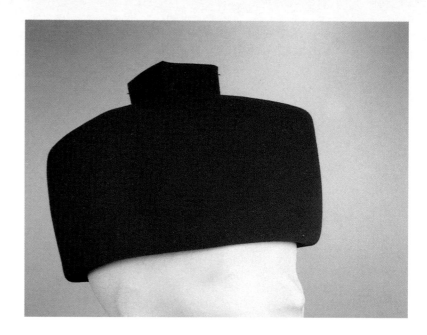

1960s red velour in a square shape, decorated with a square on top; labeled Redleaf, John Wanamaker.

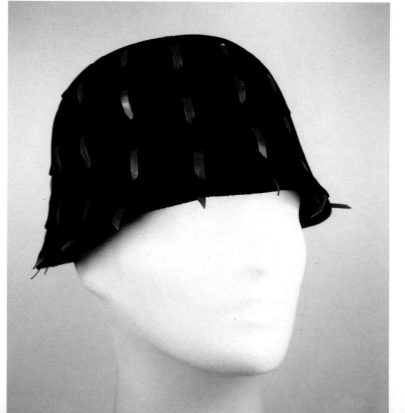

1960s tan Doeskin felt with grosgrain band veil and back feathers; labeled Designed by Sylvia, New York, St. Louis. *Courtesy of Wear It Again Sam, Manayunk.*

1960s black felt, decorated with red kid ribbons; labeled Dachettes, Designed by Lilly Daché.

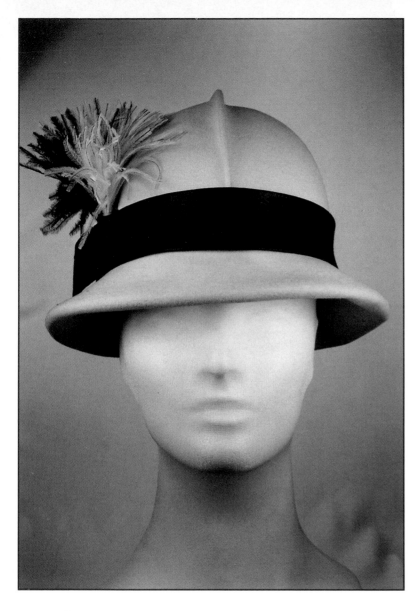

1960s off-white felt with a black kid band and feather decoration; labeled Frank Olive, New York, John Wanamaker. *Courtesy of Edna Kandle.*

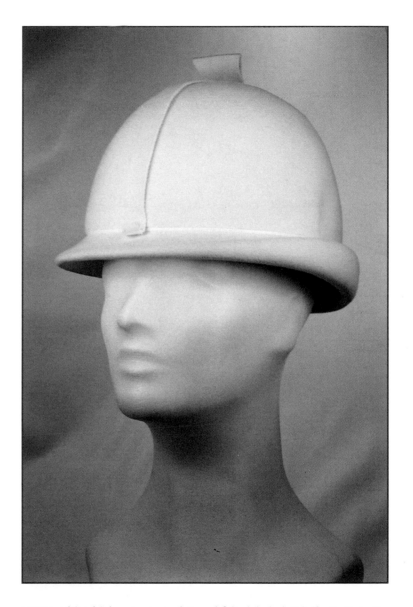

1960s white high-crown, sculptured felt; labeled Adolfo II, Paris & New York, Bonwit Teller.

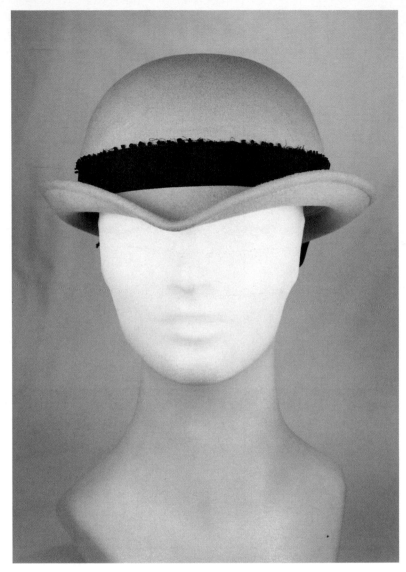

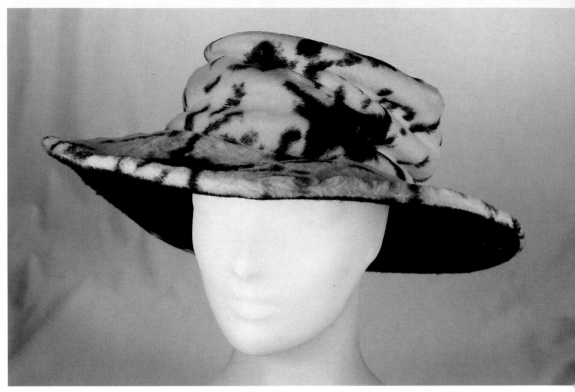

1960s floppy brim black on white velour, felt lined brim; labeled Norman Durand Original.

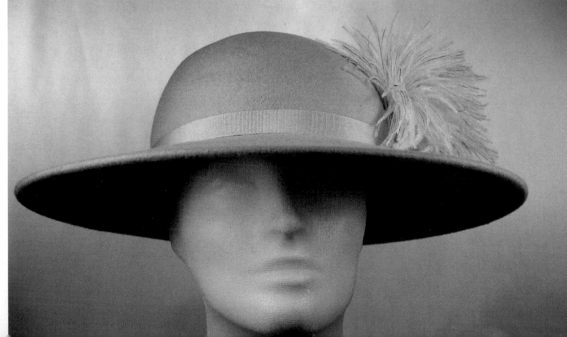

1960s felt, trimmed with black silk grosgrain ribbon; labeled Adolfo II.

Recent tan Doeskin wool felt with a shallow crown and medium-wide brim; labeled Sandra, New York, Geo. W. Bollman & Company., Inc. *Courtesy of Wear It Again Sam, Manayunk.*

❧ Horsehair ☙

Horsehair is quite literally hair fiber obtained from the mane and tail of a horse. It may be used in combination with mohair, linen, cotton, and other fibers to achieve its characteristic openwork weave. Besides widespread use in millinery, it has been used for interfacing in suits and coats, and hems in dresses and gowns.

As collectors, we are able to locate numerous mid-to-late nineteenth century horsehair hats, particularly the black horsehair mourning hats. Again very popular in the 1920s, in paler hues, for cloches and the ever popular mushroom brims, we find examples of horsehair in every decade. In the 1950s the openwork effect was virtually replaced by synthetic materials, notably nylon and acetate.

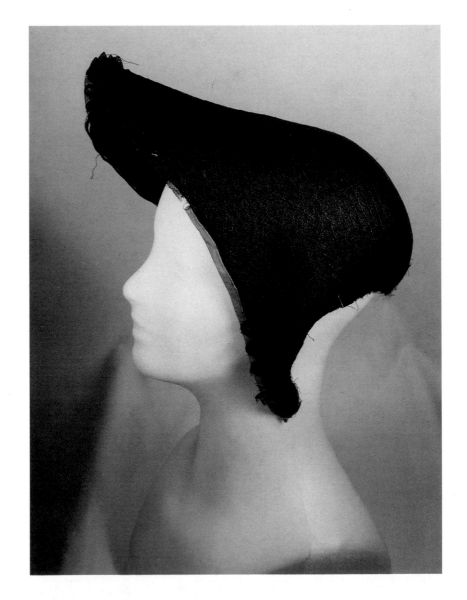

Ca. 1800 black horsehair bonnet, lined with black silk and trimmed in lilac silk.

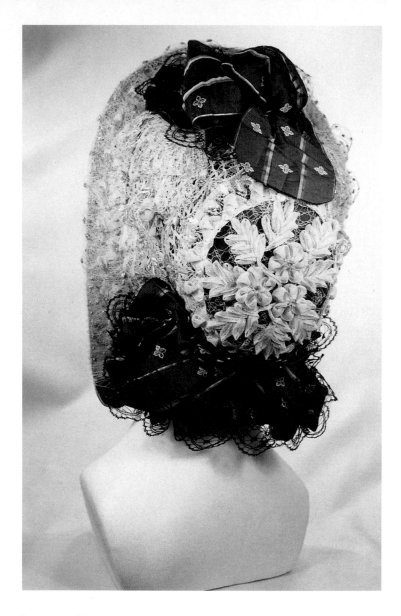

Ca. 1860 elaborately woven horsehair, covering entire outer surface of bonnet in various, intricate patterns and embroidered with fine straw, trimmed with black and green silk ribbons. *Courtesy of Karen Augusta.*

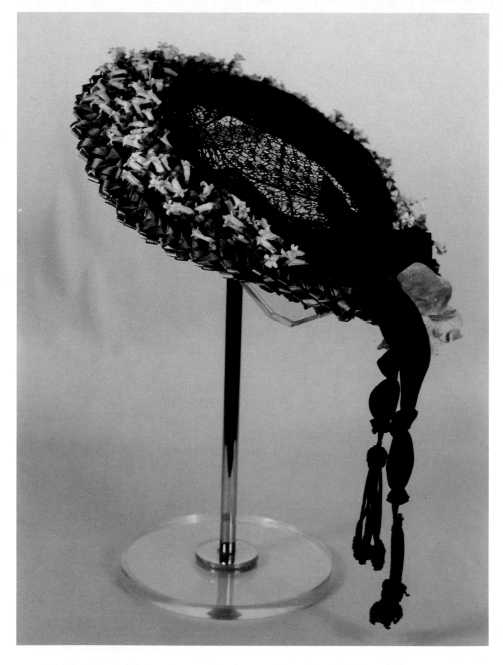

1880s horsehair bonnet on a wire frame, trimmed with silk and diminutive cloth flowers and leaves on a woven grass base; labeled Denenys, Fifth Avenue.

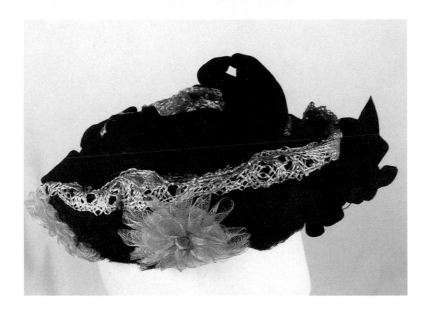

Ca. 1890 elaborately woven horsehair bonnet, trimmed with black silk velvet bows, lined with black silk; labeled Dives, Pomeroy and Stewart. *Courtesy of Alison Bartholomew.*

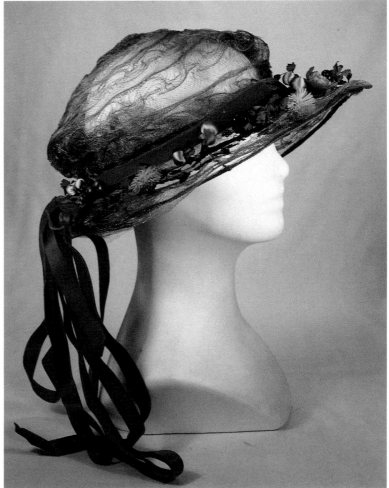

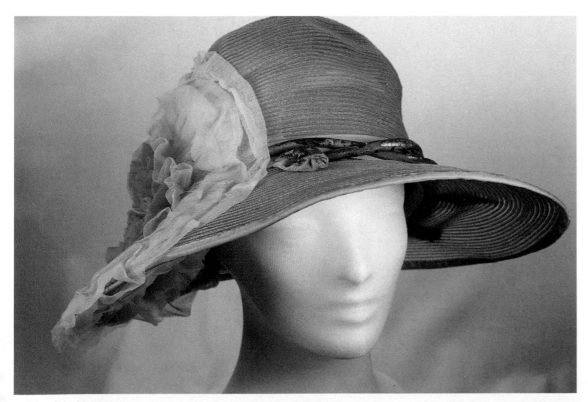

1920s horsehair on a wire frame, probably in combination with mohair, to form an open-work lace, decorated with small berries, flowers, and leaves, with an ample length of orange silk velvet ribbon. Sheer silk lining; labeled George Allen Inc., 1214 Chestnut Street, Philadelphia. Unusually vibrant and colorful. *Courtesy of Sharon Glosser.*

Ca. 1922 apricot horsehair braid with huge ombre chiffon flower on right side of hat, as well as one under right side of brim; labeled Wise, 17 E. 48th St., New York. *Courtesy of Karen Augusta.*

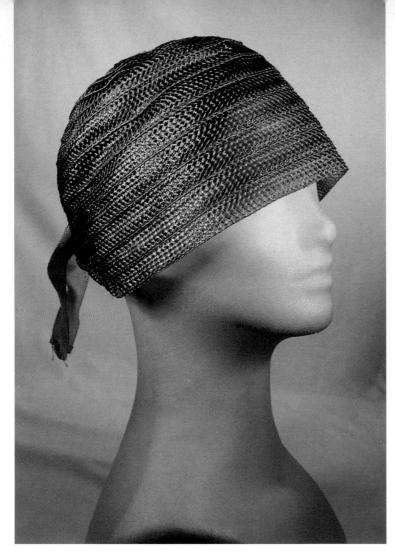

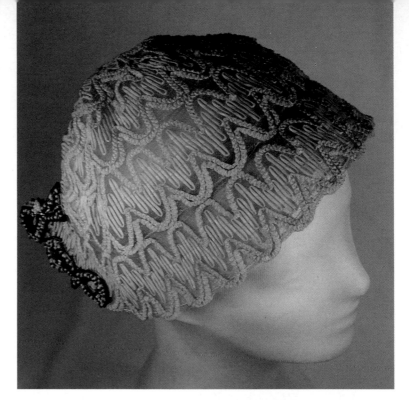

1950s horsehair, decorated with quills, trimmed with glass beads on the inside and outside of brim; labeled Peg Sturgis, Custom Millinery, 206 S. 13th St., Phila.

1920s green horsehair cloche, trimmed with a single piece of silk grosgrain ribbon, lined in silk crepe.

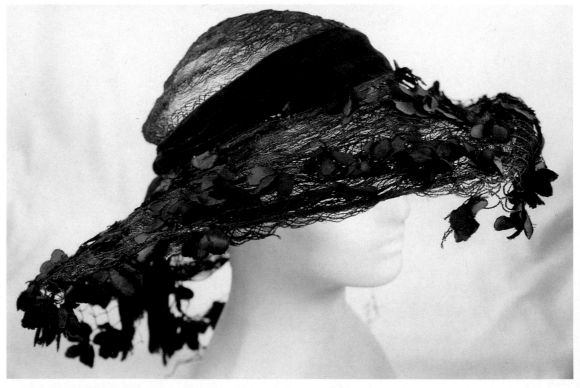

1940s black horsehair picture hat, draped in net, covered with small, silk flowers; labeled John Frederics, Made to Order; The Blum Store, Mezzanine Salon, Philadelphia.

☙ Feathers ❧

Colin McDowell, in *Hats: Status, Style and Glamour*, mentions that as early as the fourteenth century "men of rank enjoyed wearing feathers." Feathers were rare and expensive. Native American men also wore feathers as an indication of status and rank.

Although plumes were sometimes visible on the eighteenth and early nineteenth century hats for women, it was not until the last decade of the nineteenth century that extravagant display and self-adornment in millinery became commonplace. There was an extensive, if not excessive, use of feathers in millinery at this time.

McDowell mentions the case of a London feather dealer in 1892 who received a single consignment of 6,000 bird of paradise feathers, 40,000 hummingbird feathers, and 360,000 feathers from various birds in the East Indies. Large numbers of American birds were killed annually to provide for the millinery trade. We must remember that our warmer areas, such as Florida, were at one time inhabited by many species of exotic birds.

In 1885, a bill was passed in New Jersey forbidding the killing of any bird not generally known as a game bird. The guiding principle of the Audubon Society, formed at this time, was the prevention of the wearing of feathers as ornaments, or trimming for dress. In other words, the Audubon Society provided for the preservation of exotic birds.

Some feathers were considered acceptable, such as those from domestic birds, geese, ducks, cockerels, pheasants, and ostriches. An ostrich can be plucked without harming the bird. This, we hope, accounts for the large number of ostrich feathers used in millinery.

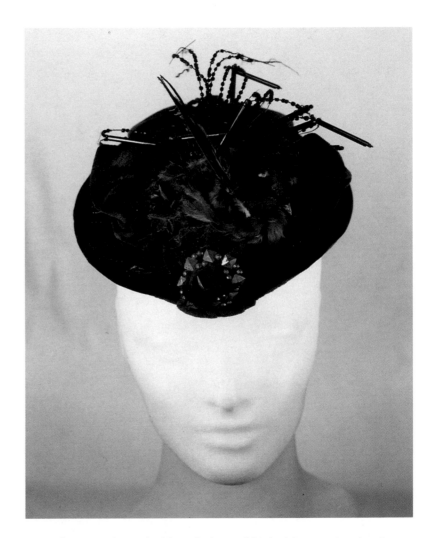

1890s bonnet, trimmed with a whole small bird, elaborate glass beading and velvet ruching. *Courtesy of Alison Bartholomew.*

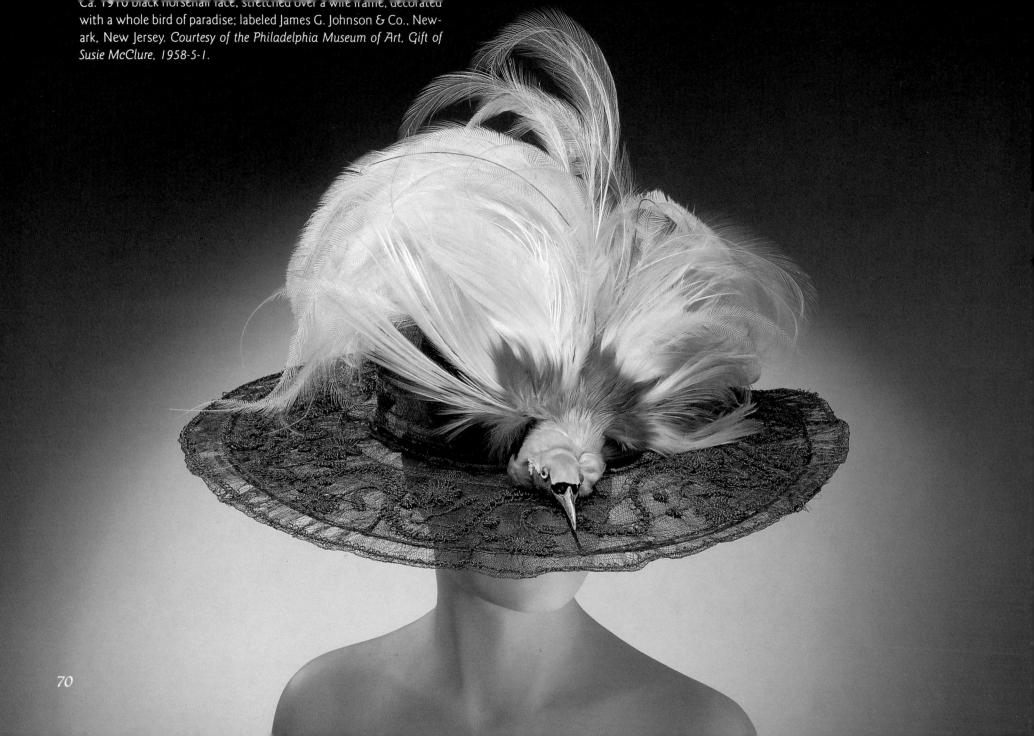

Ca. 1910 black horsehair lace, stretched over a wire frame, decorated with a whole bird of paradise; labeled James G. Johnson & Co., Newark, New Jersey. *Courtesy of the Philadelphia Museum of Art. Gift of Susie McClure, 1958-5-1.*

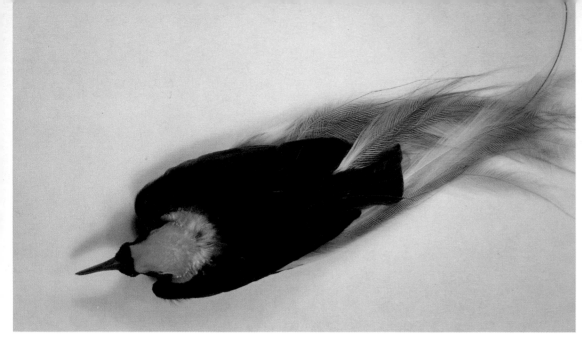

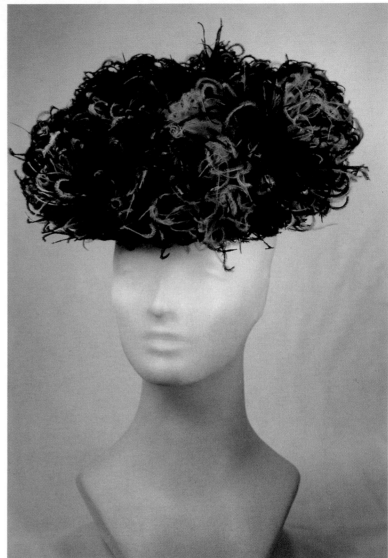

Ca. 1900 full bird of paradise, taken off a hat "seventy-nine years ago." *Courtesy of Katherine Stauffer.*

Ca. 1900 full bird of paradise, taken off a hat "seventy-nine years ago." *Courtesy of Katherine Stauffer.* This whole bird and the one previously pictured were taken off hats that belonged to Mrs. Stauffer's mother.

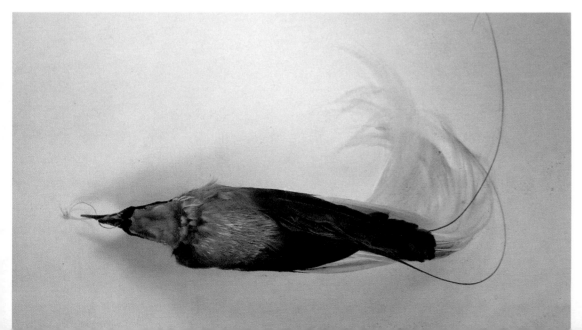

1930s "doll hat," covered with aqua and black ostrich feathers; labeled John B. Stetson, 1224 Chestnut Street, Philadelphia. *Acquired from Elizabeth A. Freame.*

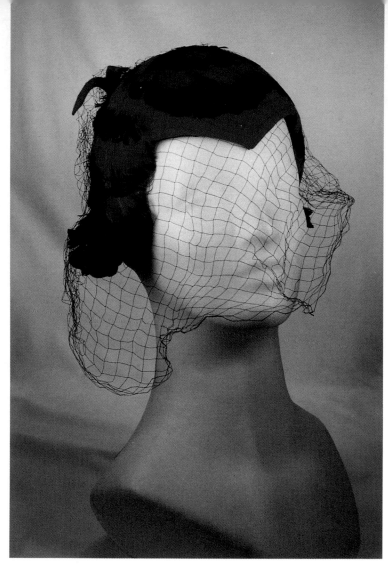

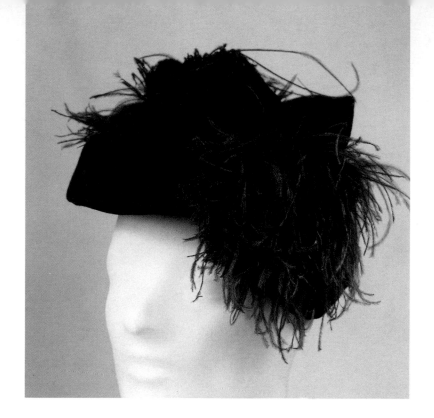

1930s blue felt with dyed ostrich feathers above and below the brim.

1930s fuchsia and black feather helmet, lined with black silk; labeled Hattie Carnegie Original, Chertak, Walnut at 17th, Philadelphia. *Acquired from Elizabeth A. Freame.* The helmet style is most unusual in a feather decorated fashion hat.

1940s black shiny straw, with horsehair overlay and pink and green feather trim designed to resemble flowers; labeled Rubin, New York.

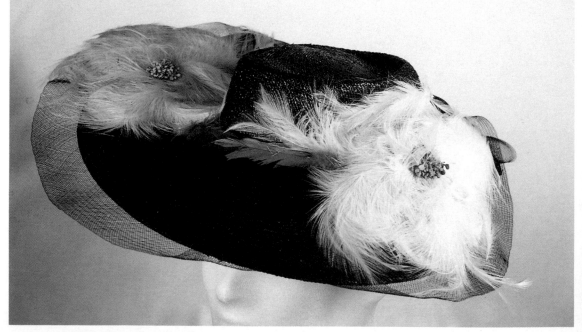

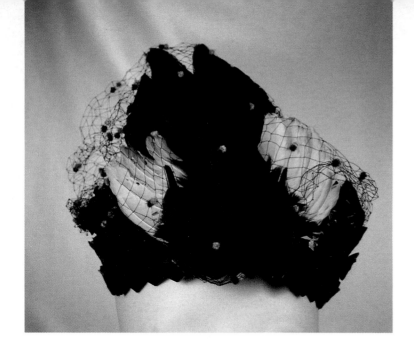

1940s navy cellophane straw with navy and white birds, with black celluloid beaks, original hatpins, chenille dotted veil; labeled Custom Made Laddie Northridge, 1 W. 57th St., New York. *Acquired from Elizabeth A. Freame.*

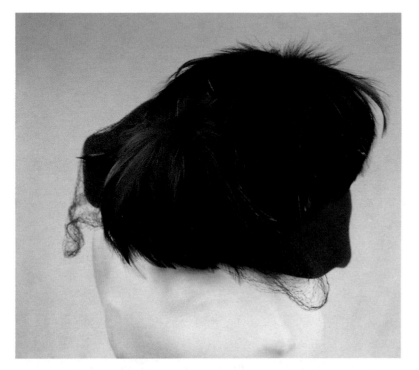

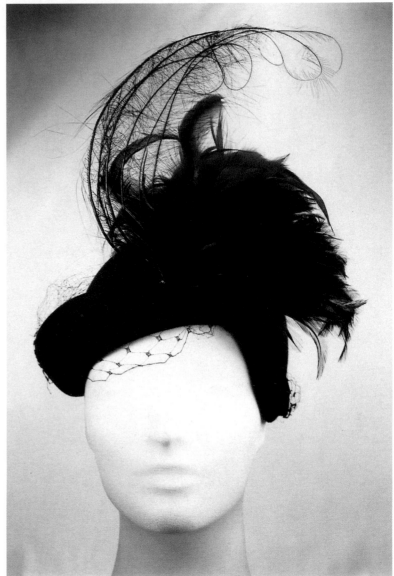

1940s black "hand finished" fur felt, with veil and brown and black feathers; labeled Vogue, 27 East State St., Trenton, New Jersey.

1940s "scottie" type velour with elaborate dyed feather detailing.

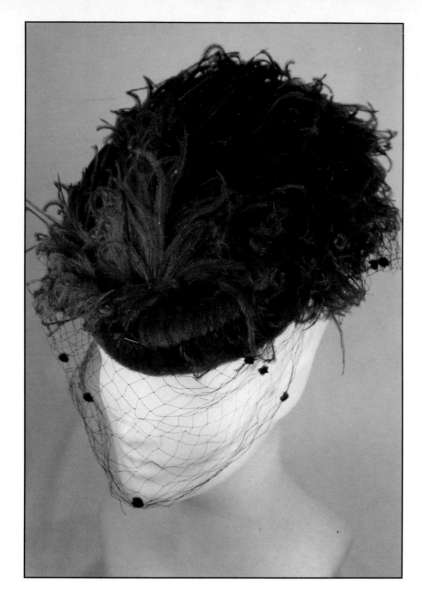

1940s burnt orange ostrich feathers, trimmed with satin ribbon and chenille dotted veil; labeled Nancy Bee, Stylist, 385 Bridge St., Brooklyn.

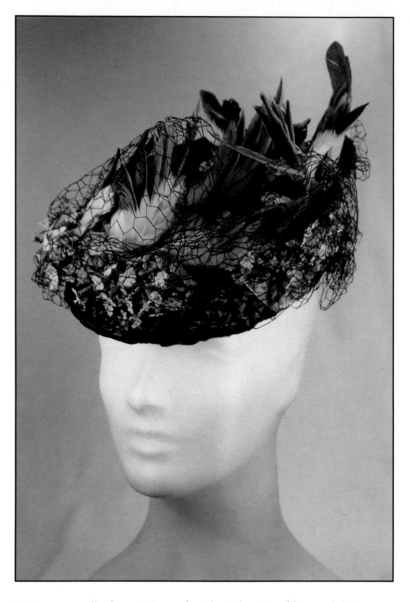

1940s navy cellophane, trimmed with pink satin ribbon, miniature pale blue flowers, upswept bird's wings in shades of pink and rose; labeled Custom Made Laddie Northridge, Inc., 1 W. 57th St., New York.

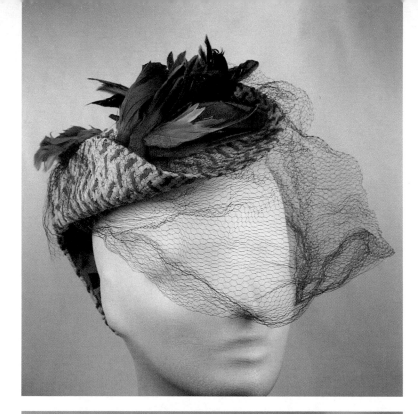

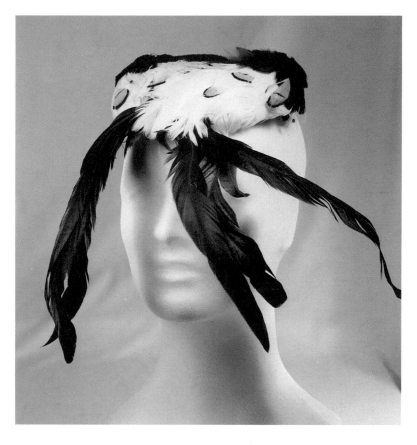

1940s pink and green cellophane straw with rose and green upswept feathers, to resemble birds in flight, veil; labeled Laddie Northridge, 14 W. 57th St., New York.

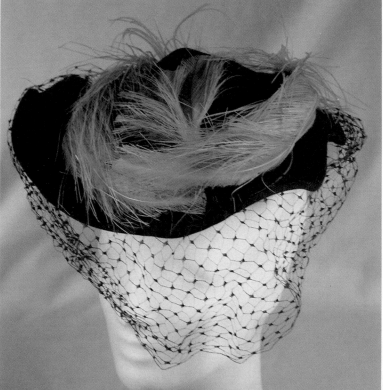

1940s "doll hat" decorated with cloth daisies and feathers that partially cover the face; labeled Hattie Carnegie. *Courtesy of the Drexel Historic Costume Collection, Nesbitt College of Design Arts, Drexel University.*

1940s purple felt with chartreuse feathers; labeled Nan Duskin. *Courtesy of the Drexel Historic Costume Collection, Nesbitt College of Design Arts, Drexel University.*

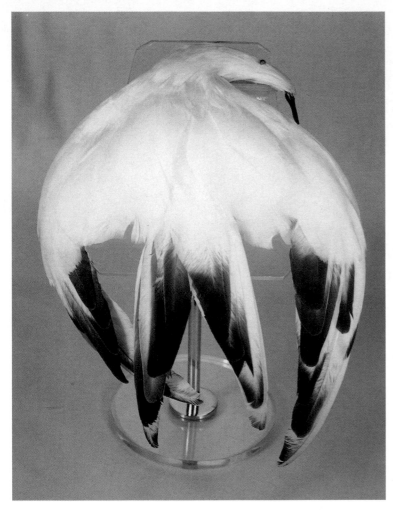

1940s millinery bird, made up of feathers, glued on a white gauze pattern; glass eyes, celluloid beak; labeled Paris, No. 888, Made In France. *Acquired from Elizabeth A. Freame.*

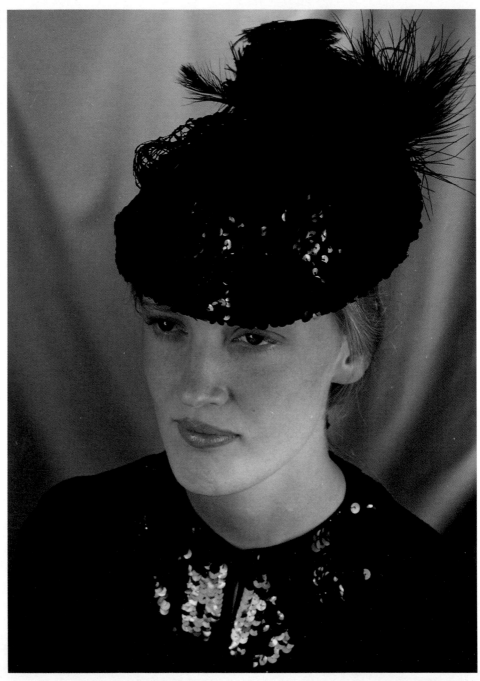

1940s black sequins and feathers on a stiffened net base. *Modeled by Marcie Behanna.*

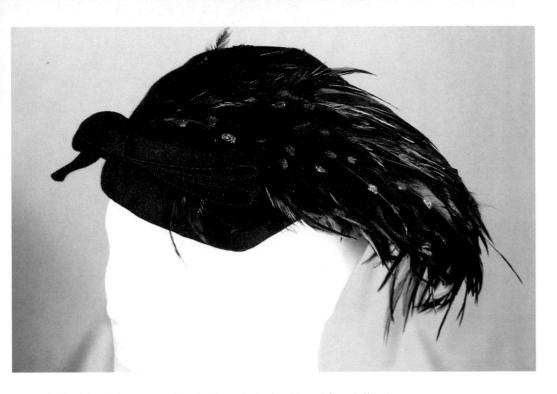

1940s felt with a sweeping feather, dotted with gold metallic; labeled Stewart & Co., Baltimore.

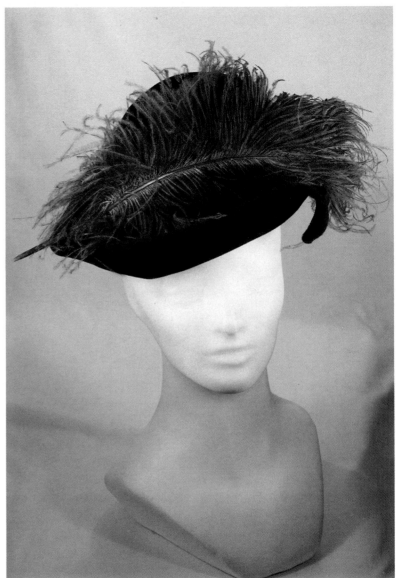

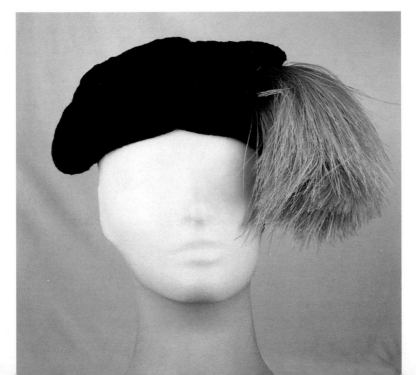

1940s burgundy velour a with burgundy tinted ostrich feather.

1940s black braided felt with a pink feather; labeled Milgrim.

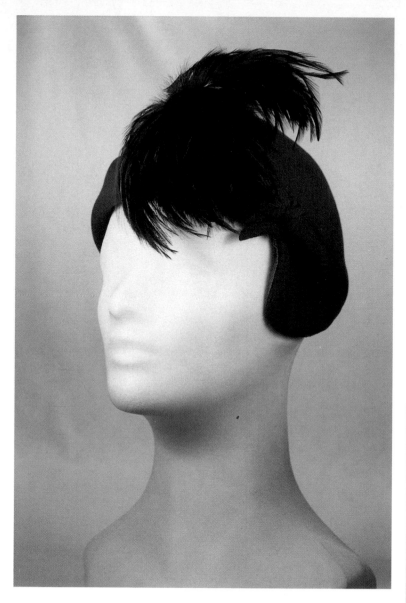

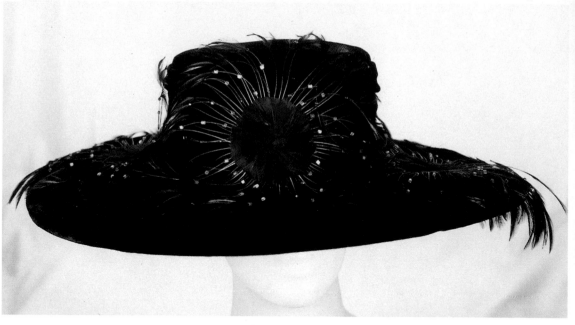

1950s wide brimmed velvet, decorated with stripped and beaded feathers.

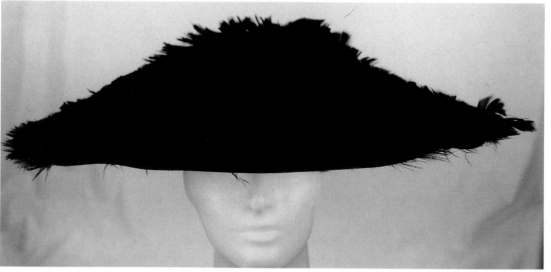

1940s "helmet" style velour with a stand up feather.

1950s wide brim, entirely covered with black feathers, crown and underside of brim in fur felt; labeled originals by Fló-Raye, New York.

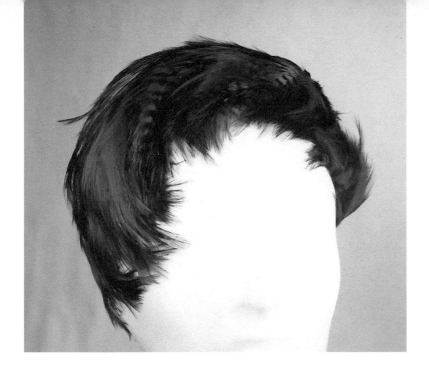

1950s green feather clip.

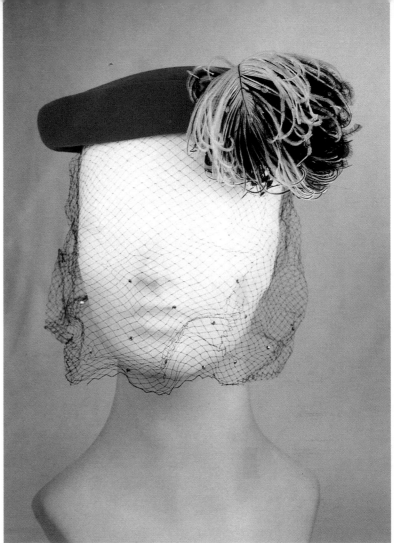

1950s red velvet with contrasting feather and rhinestone dotted veil.

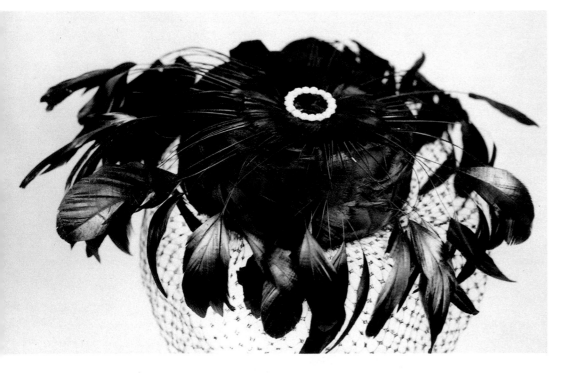

1960s black feather covered pillbox, veil is attached with a rhinestone circle at center of crown.

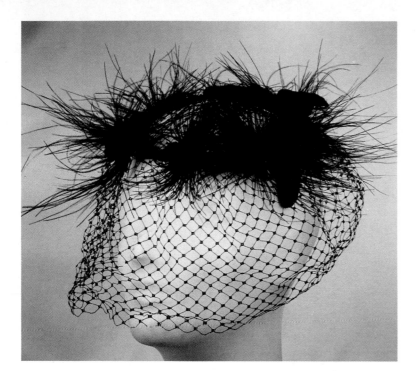

1960s net "cage" hat decorated with feathers to resemble flowers.

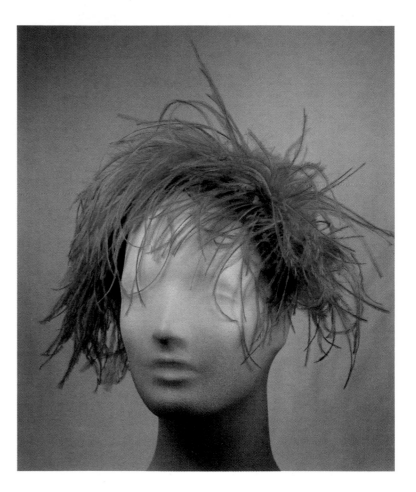

1960s blue ostrich feather headband; labeled J Jrs.

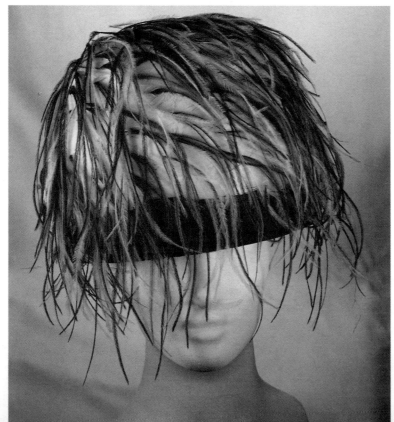

1960s white velour with pink velvet visor, high crown completely decorated with feathers in several layers; labeled Don Anderson, New York.

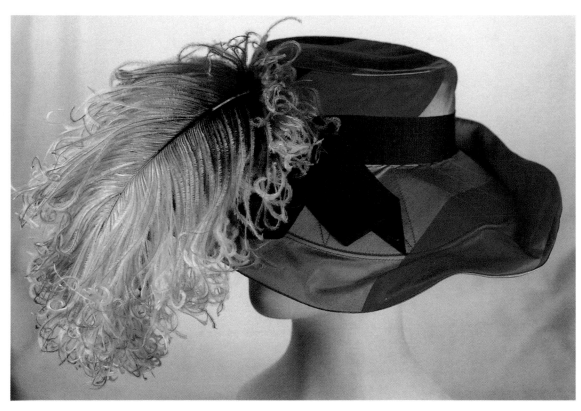

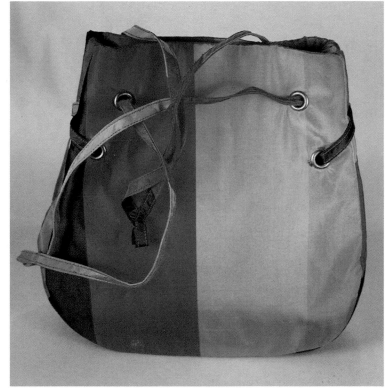

1960s taffeta in shades of plum, pink, and rose, ostrich plume in
chartreuse and orange, plum grosgrain band; labeled Norman Durand
Original.

Pink taffeta pocketbook; labeled Sherman. Saint Louis, matches the
Durand hat.

ꙮ Silk ꙮ

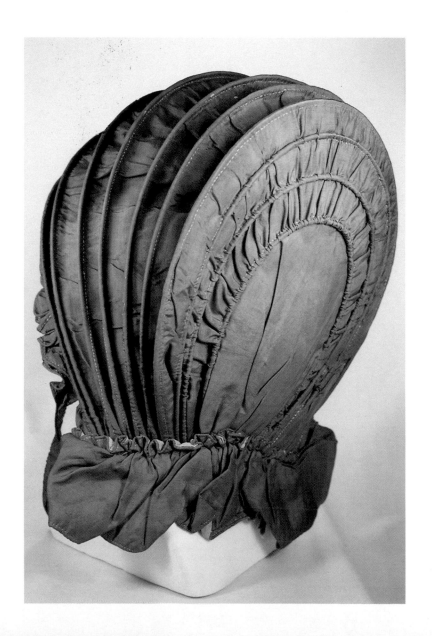

1810 brown silk calash lined with gauze, a very early hat with excellent provenance. *Courtesy of Alison Bartholomew.*

Silk, satin, rayon, and nylon are all used in millinery.

Pure silk has a long history of lining and trimming millinery. It was also a primary material for making hats and bonnets, but is so susceptible to heat and moisture damage that fewer of these early, entirely silk bonnets and hats have survived than the more durable felts and straws.

Traditionally expensive because it must be imported from the Orient, silk is fiber from the cocoon of the silkworm. Although known as a strong fabric, we value it especially because it is sheer, smooth, and luxurious.

Rayon was originally known as artificial silk. It is a fiber derived from trees, cotton, and woody plants. According to *Fairchild's Dictionary of Fashion*, it was first produced by Count Hilaire de Chardonet in 1889, and it was worn at Queen Victoria's funeral in 1901. Much less costly than silk, rayon has a shiny, lustrous appearance and good draping quality. This quality of draping well makes it ideal for millinery.

Satin is not a textile, but rather a type of finish used on various textiles such as silk, rayon, acetate, nylon, or combinations of these yarns. Popular in millinery because it is so lustrous and smooth, a satin finish often makes it difficult to discern the actual textile used.

Acetate is a generic term for fiber artificially made from cellulose acetate. Acetate drapes well and has a silk-like appearance, but it tends to turn purplish with age.

Nylon is a generic term for artificial fiber made of a long chain of synthetic polyamides extracted from coal and petroleum. According to *Fairchild's Dictionary of Fashion*, it was introduced in 1939 by Dupont and later produced by other manufacturers. Nylon can be washed, and it is resistant to mildew and moths. It was used extensively in 1950s millinery.

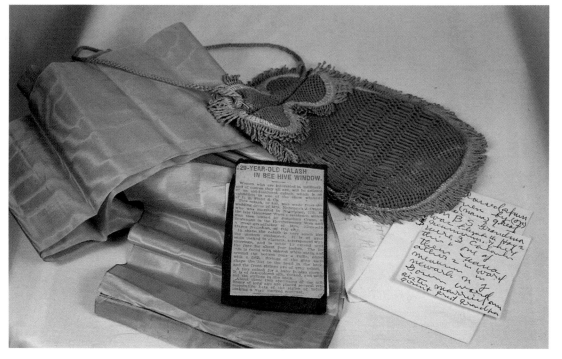

Documentation relating to the 1810 calash (pictured). Pocketbook and wide silk sash were worn during 1798 wedding ceremony.

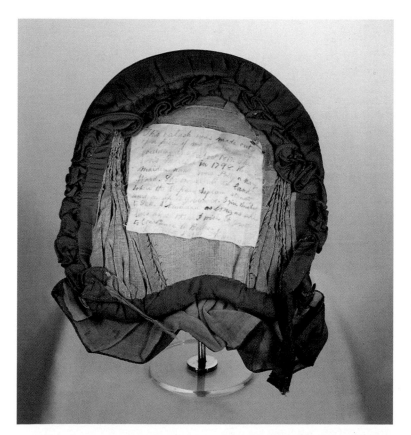

Verbatim from cloth inside hat (pictured): "This calash was made out of a piece of my grandmother Grimes wedding dress about 1810. She was married in 1798. Her maiden name was Polly or Mary Ward. She owned all the land where the Orphan Asylum stands and on up to Golden St. I give this hat to Stella A. Neumann as long as she lives and then I wish to give it to Constance O. Bolles. S. Elizabeth Hayes Neumann."

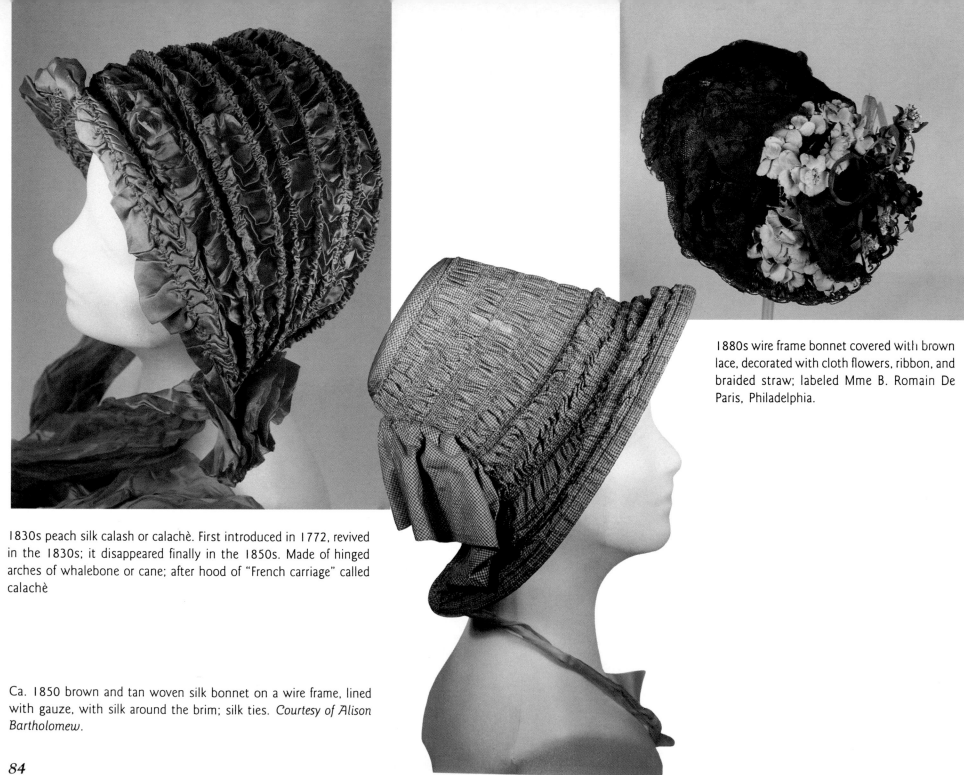

1880s wire frame bonnet covered with brown lace, decorated with cloth flowers, ribbon, and braided straw; labeled Mme B. Romain De Paris, Philadelphia.

1830s peach silk calash or calachè. First introduced in 1772, revived in the 1830s; it disappeared finally in the 1850s. Made of hinged arches of whalebone or cane; after hood of "French carriage" called calachè

Ca. 1850 brown and tan woven silk bonnet on a wire frame, lined with gauze, with silk around the brim; silk ties. *Courtesy of Alison Bartholomew.*

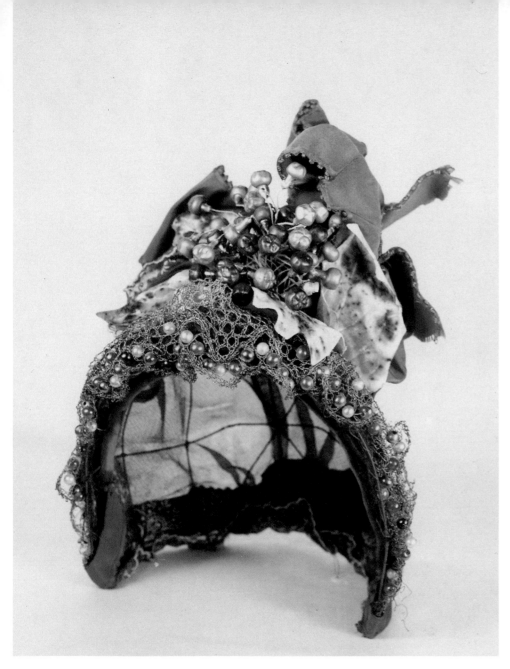

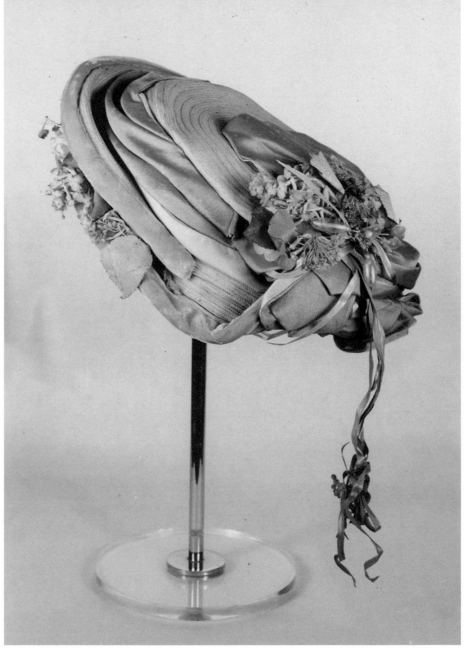

Ca. 1880 silk bonnet on a wire frame detailing of hand embroidered silk chiffon, silk ribbon, silk velvet, tulle, hand painted silk velvet leaves, and pearls in burgundy, white and gray, stand up glass beads in tan and black, Birkenbine Estate.

1880s straw bonnet interspersed with silk ribbon, cloth flowers, velvet, and glass beads, inner-brim is constructed of tucks of straw and silk, lined in eggshell silk; labeled Adolph Heller, Paris Millinery, 21 North Eighth St., Philadelphia.

1890s silk bonnet, trimmed with black sequins and a feather; labeled Lillias Hurd, 326 Fifth Avenue, New York. *Courtesy of the Drexel Historic Costume Collection, Nesbitt College of Design Arts, Drexel University.*

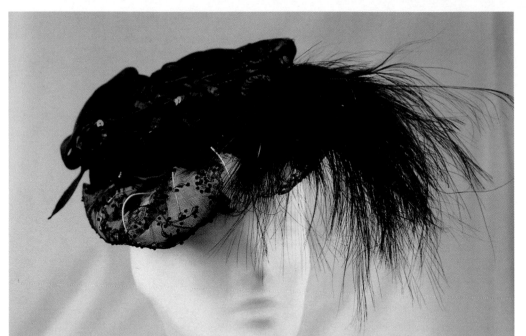

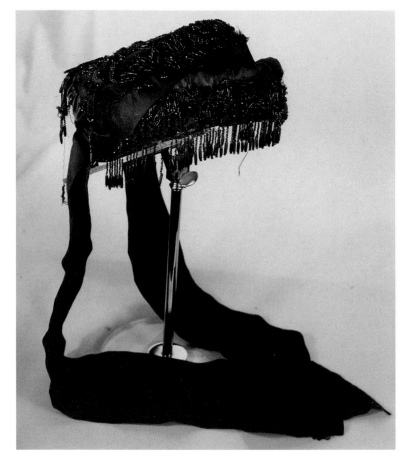

Ca. 1890 blue silk bonnet, trimmed with black and blue beads on net, with an intricate fringe of beads around hat, wide silk ties, lined with black silk, Birkenbine Estates.

Ca. 1900 wide brimmed paisley silk in shacks of yellow and tan, with an underbrim of green silk velvet and trimmed with green and blue, iridescent sequins and green silk velvet ribbon. *Courtesy of Alison Bartholomew.*

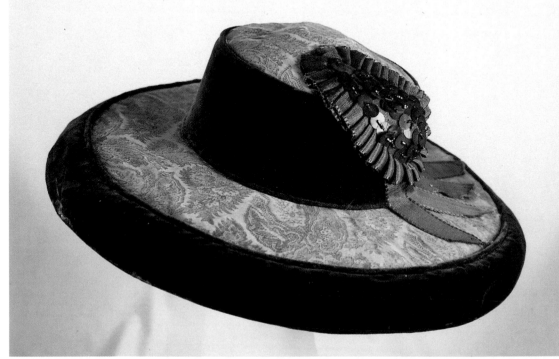

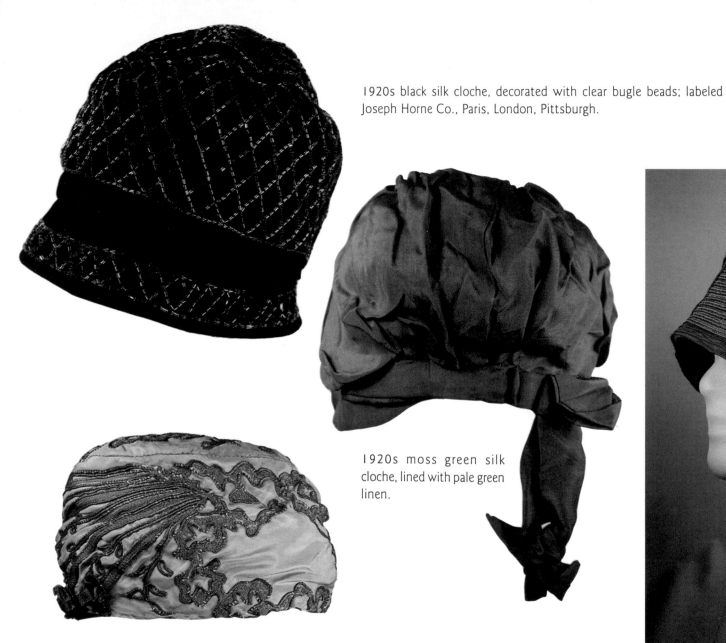

1920s black silk cloche, decorated with clear bugle beads; labeled Joseph Horne Co., Paris, London, Pittsburgh.

1920s moss green silk cloche, lined with pale green linen.

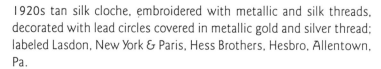

1920s tan silk cloche, embroidered with metallic and silk threads, decorated with lead circles covered in metallic gold and silver thread; labeled Lasdon, New York & Paris, Hess Brothers, Hesbro, Allentown, Pa.

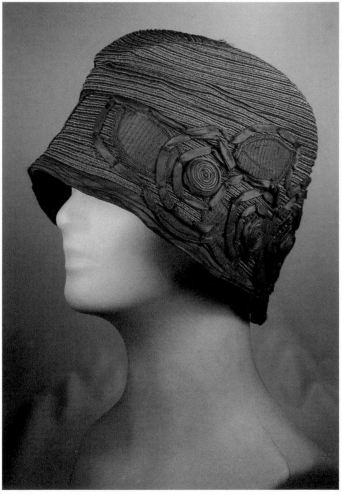

1920s mauve silk toque, decorated in same-color silk ribbon, floral patterns; labeled FMC Caprice, Paris & New York. *Gift from Margaret Heath Smith.*

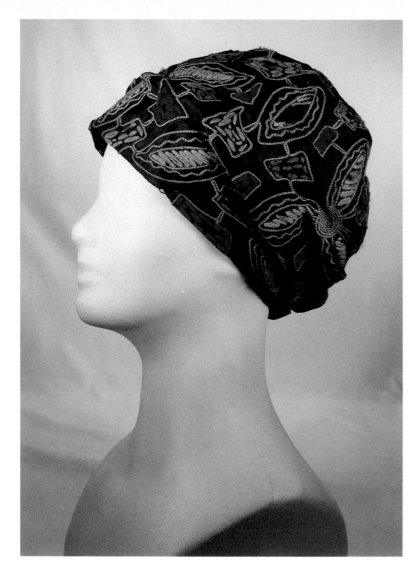

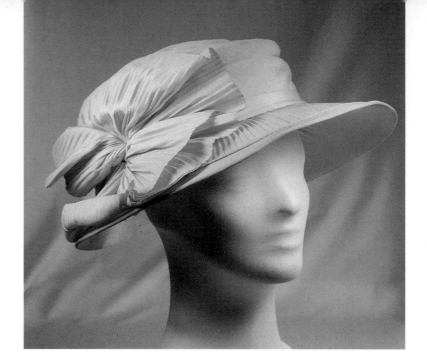

1920s mushroom brim, softly draped with eggshell pleated silk. *Courtesy of the Drexel Historic Costume Collection, Nesbitt College of Design Arts, Drexel University.*

1920s brown silk cloche, embroidered with gold braid and red, light green, and turquoise wool; labeled Tailored Hats. Phipps, London, Paris, New York, Geo. M. Keebler, 1428 Chestnut St., Philadelphia.

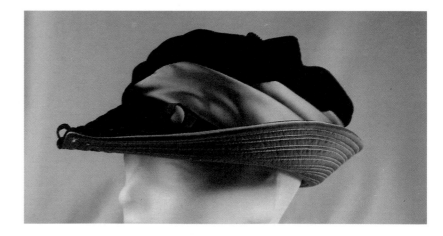

1920s black velvet and lilac silk cloche, trimmed with silk ribbon, soft brim; labeled Naiman's Mirror Fashions, 1020 Chestnut Street, Philadelphia. *Courtesy of the Drexel Historic Costume Collection, Nesbitt College of Design Arts, Drexel University.*

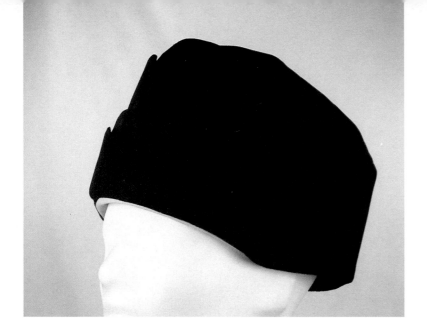

1920s silk crepe toque, lined with white silk; labeled The Mourning Shop, 1835 Chestnut Street, Philadelphia.

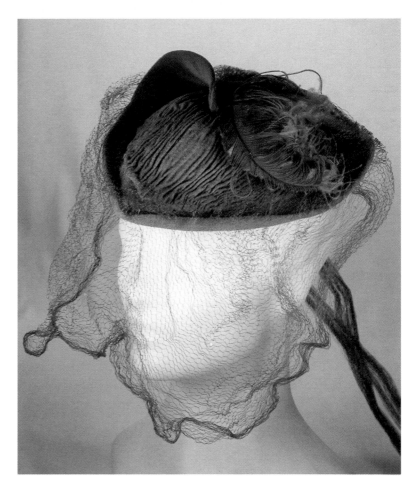

1930s silk crepe, detailed with tucks, veil, feathers, and streamers. Beautifully constructed.

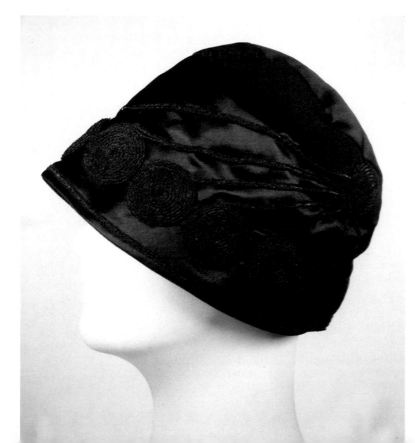

1920s silk satin cloche, appliquéd with black straw in circular stitched patterns; labeled Gimbel Brothers, Philadelphia, New York, Paris.

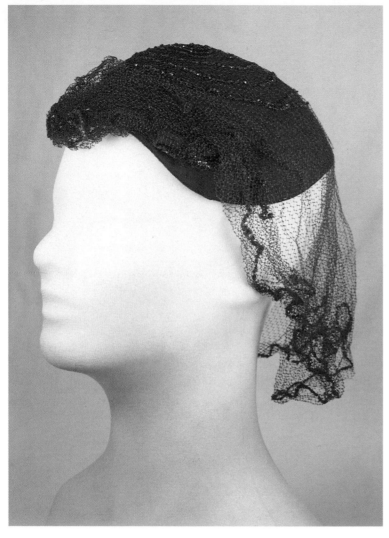

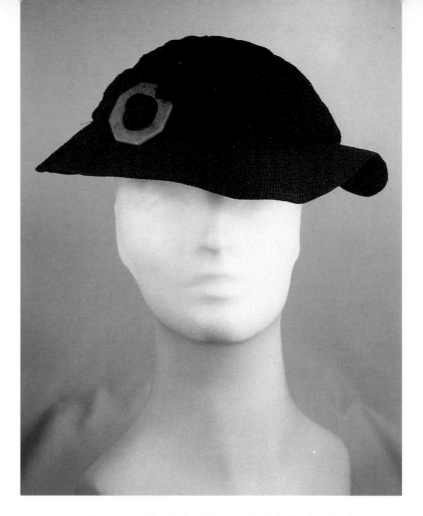

1930s navy silk crepe with stitched brim and a bakelite buckle decoration.

1930s green silk, decorated with clear bugle beads and elaborate, all-over veil which hangs behind hat and is also beaded.

1940s black silk organza, draped over a quilted brim and crown, trimmed with wide fuchsia silk ribbon; labeled G. Howard Hodge, Seven Eleven Fifth Avenue, New York, registered model. A fascinating hat because of its large size and exquisite materials.

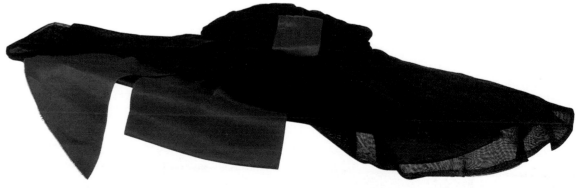

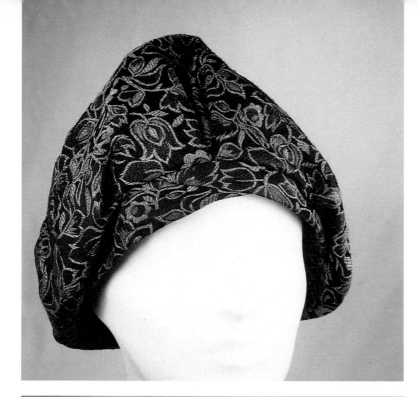

1950s black and gold brocade turban.

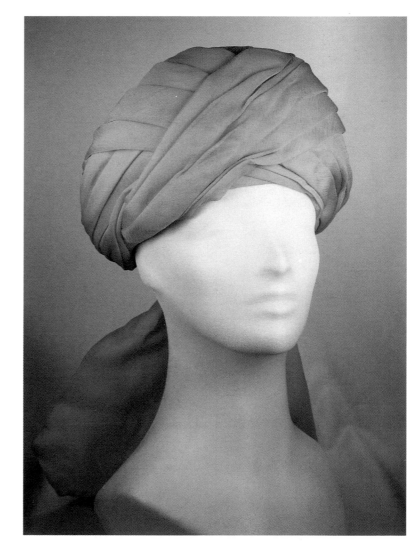

1950s silk chiffon open-crown turban; labeled Irene of New York, Lord & Taylor Salon.

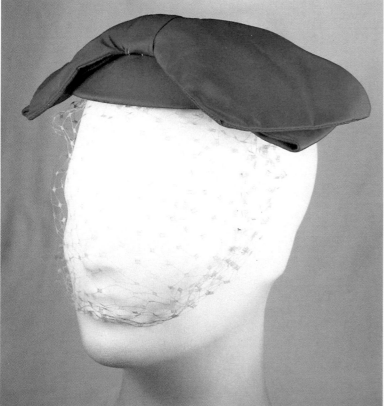

1950s green silk cocktail hat, large bow and pale green veil; labeled Mr. D, Hess Brothers, Allentown, Pa.

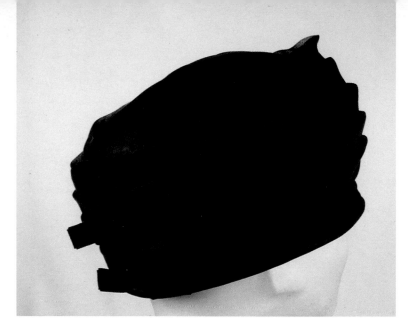

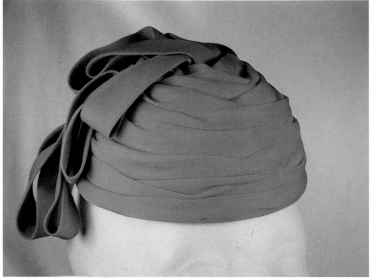

1960s turquoise silk "doll hat"; labeled Miss Sally Victor, New York. Very likely this was redesigned from a 1940s style, since the "doll hats" were popular in the 1930s and '40s, but the Miss Sally Victor label was not used until 1962.

1960s black silk organdy, trimmed with velvet bows; labeled Miss Carnegie by Hattie Carnegie.

1960s green rayon satin pillbox, decorated with three green feathers, veil.

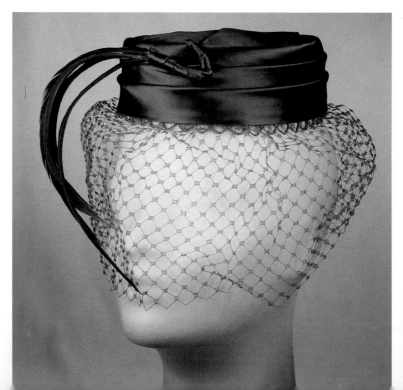

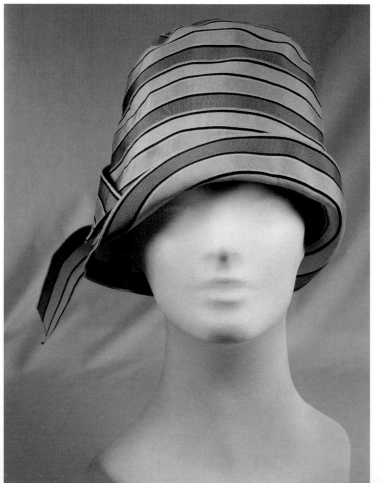

1960s yellow and tan grosgrain ribbon silk toque; labeled Mr. John, Bonwit Teller. *Courtesy of the Drexel Historic Costume Collection, Nesbitt College of Design Arts, Drexel University.*

❧ Velvet ❧

Velvet is a pile fabric, which is what gives it its thick, soft texture . It is made of various fibers in different weights, woven with an extra yarn in the warp. In a pile fabric such as terry cloth, the loops are visible. In velvet, the loops have been cut. Corduroy and velveteen are cut pile also.

Most of the nineteenth and early twentieth century velvet is made of silk pile. Many early straw bonnets are trimmed with silk velvet, and a few examples still exist that are made entirely of silk velvet.

As a primary fabric, and as a trim, velvet has been a favorite with milliners. During the 1930s, rayon velvet became popular because it cost less to produce. In the 1950s and 1960s, much of the velvet used in millinery was made of cotton and synthetic fibers.

In the last five years, rayon velvet has again become popular for millinery. Silk velvet is rarely used, except as trim on the most expensive, custom designed hats.

Ca. 1890 silk velvet bonnet, trimmed with grosgrain silk ribbon, lined with black silk; labeled Miss C. McLaughlin, Millinery Parlor, 226 Armat Street, Germantown.

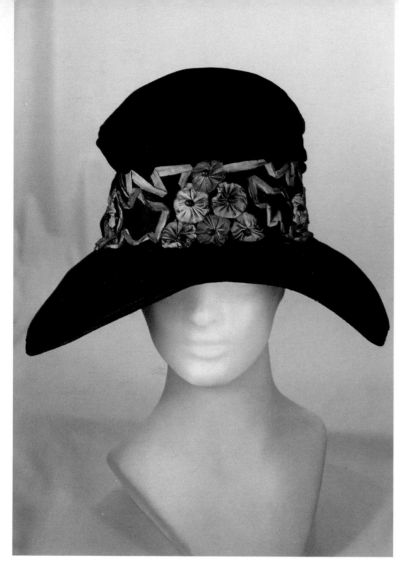

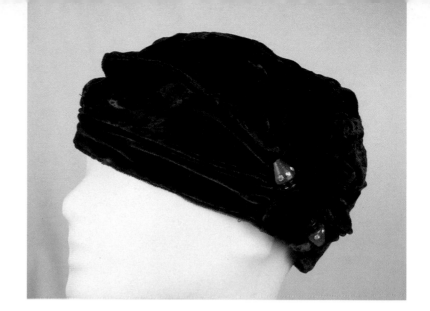

1920s brown silk velvet cloche with bakelite and rhinestone hatpin.

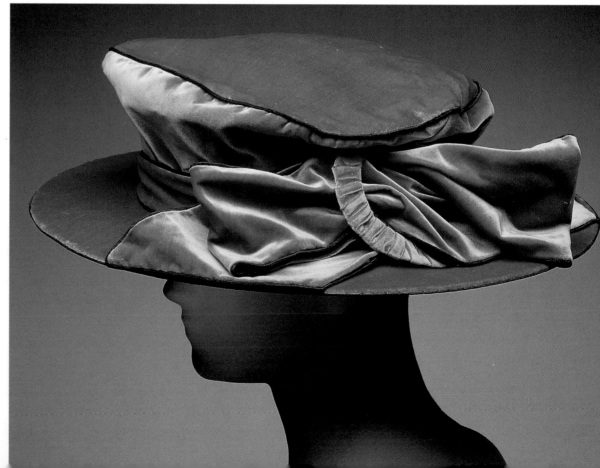

Ca. 1910 black silk velvet bonnet, lined with orange silk satin; decorated with green and orange painted ribbon and pinwheels, dotted with wooden beads.

Ca. 1917 burnt orange and black silk velvet, with a high, soft crown, wide brim and over-sized bow; Joseph G. Darlington & Company, Chestnut Street, Philadelphia. *Courtesy of the Philadelphia Museum of Art. Gift of Constance A. and Adelaide S. Jones, 1972-178-16.*

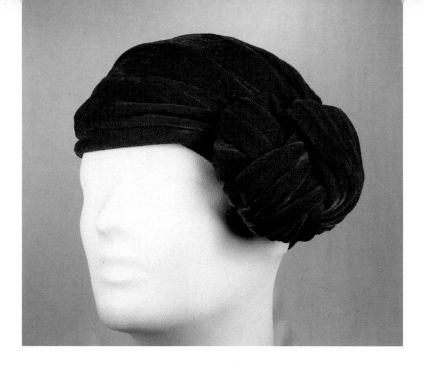

1920s purple silk velvet cloche, "knot-like" side decoration, made of 12 separate pieces.

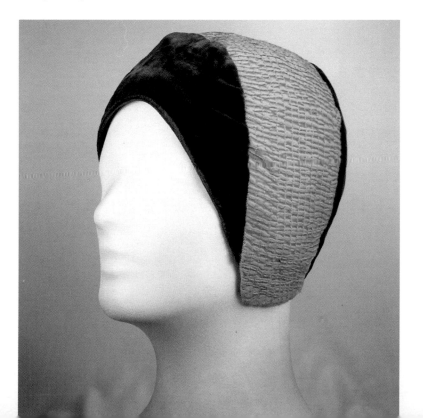

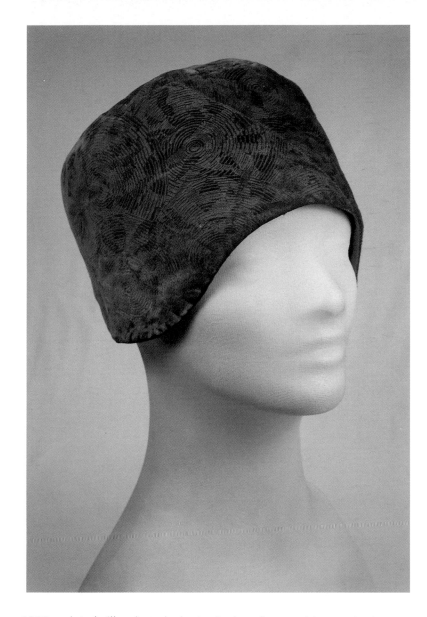

1920s printed silk velvet cloche in shades of tan and burgundy; labeled Jay Hat, Paris & New York.

1920s brown silk velvet cloche, decorated with tan smocked silk.

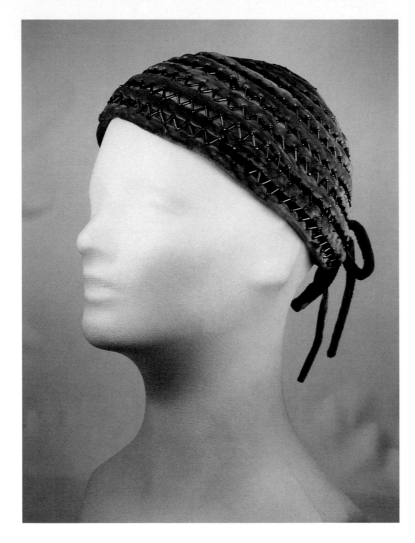

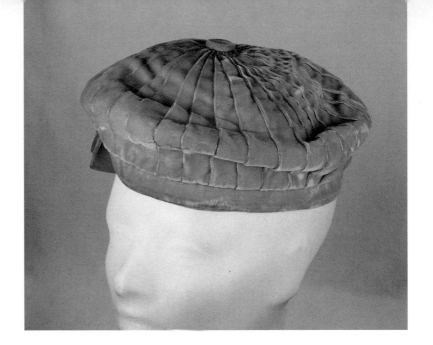

1930s silk velvet beret, made of ribbon stitched together and radiating from single covered button on crown, lace lined; labeled Reproduction of Original Gilbert Orcel, Paris.

1930s tan silk velvet ribbon, wrapped in a circular manner and attached together with copper bugle beads; labeled Hattie Carnegie Original, The Blum Store, Philadelphia.

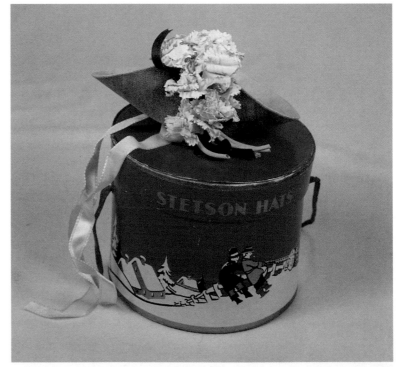

1930s miniature pale green velvet Stetson, with a cloth flower, perched on its original holiday box. *Acquired from Katherine Stauffer.*

1930s green silk velvet, trimmed with green dyed feathers and veil.

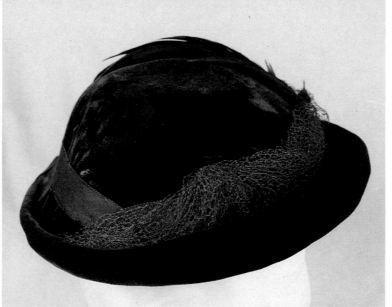

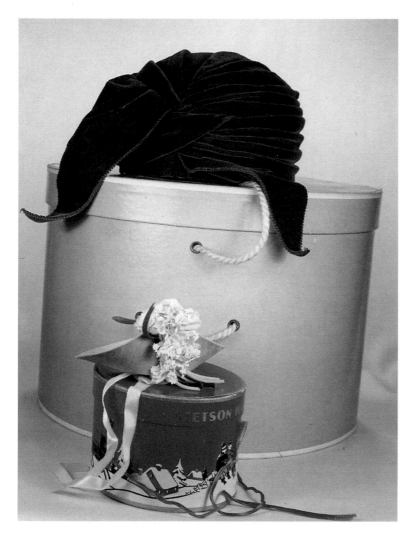

1940s teal blue silk velvet turban; labeled Miss Alice, Lord & Taylor.
Shown with miniature Stetson.

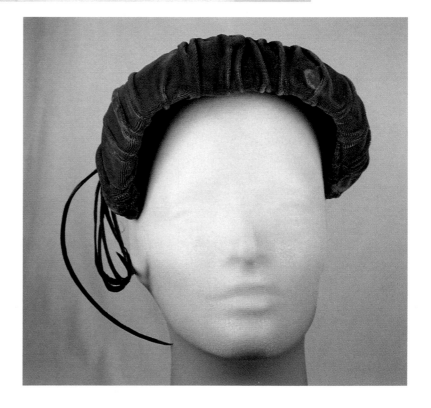

1930s green silk velvet, clip style with ruffled edge.

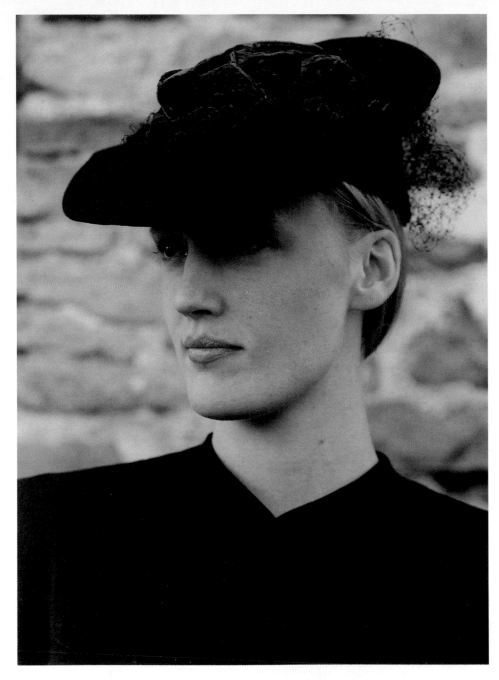

1930s black felt with blue velveteen flowers and veil; labeled
Bowman's Harrisburg, Pa. *Modeled by Marcie Behanna.*

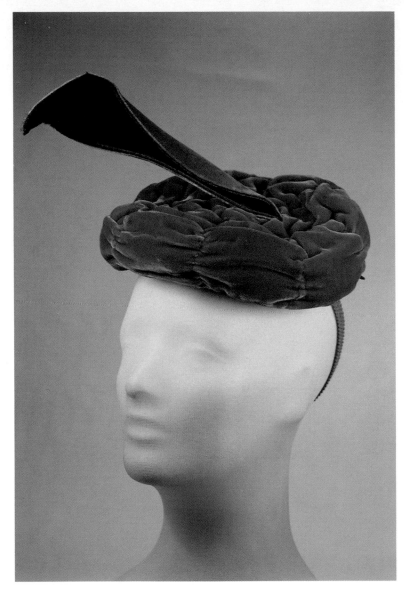

1930s rose silk velvet gathered with velvet and velour "feather" inspired decoration in shades of rose and purple.

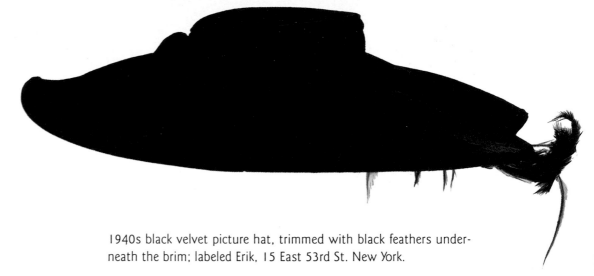

1940s black velvet picture hat, trimmed with black feathers underneath the brim; labeled Erik, 15 East 53rd St. New York.

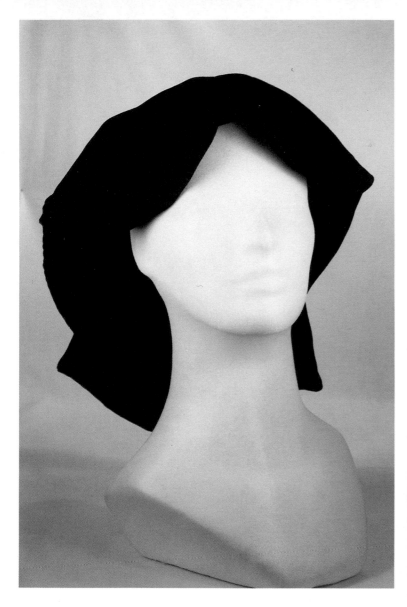

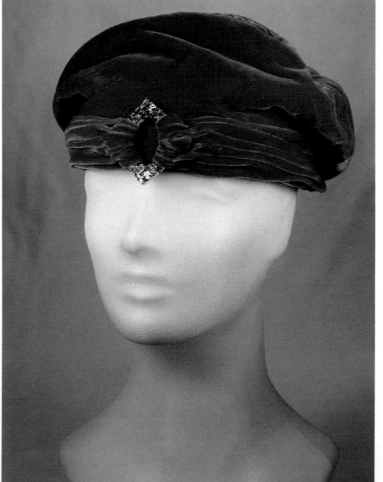

1940s deep purple silk velvet drape, beautifully designed to fall to the shoulders from a simple band of silk velvet; labeled Adrian Original, Julius Garfincket & Co., Washington. *Acquired from Ivana Tyler.* Hats designed by Adrian are rare, and are highly prized by collectors.

1940s peach velvet with rhinestone buckle in front, lined with silk crepe; labeled Emme, Bonwit Teller.

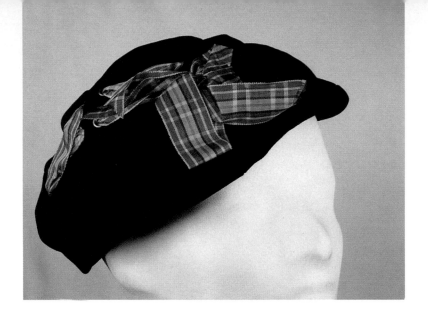

1940s black velveteen cap, with plaid taffeta laced through metal eyelets.

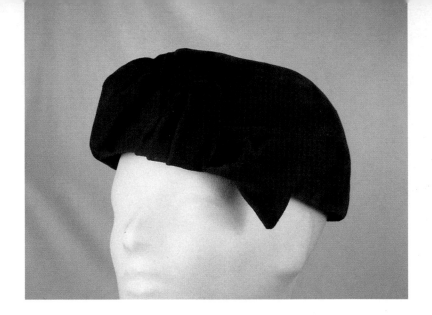

1940s plum silk velvet hat; labeled Ryder's , 4862-64 N. Broad St., Philadelphia.

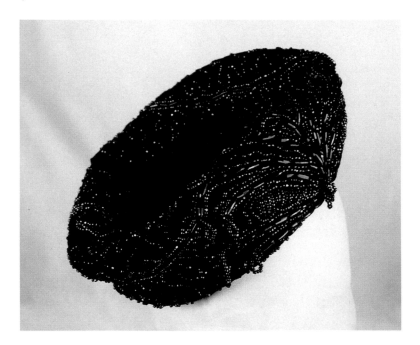

1940s black beaded velvet, intricate bead work, some beads are designed to hang from upswept brim.

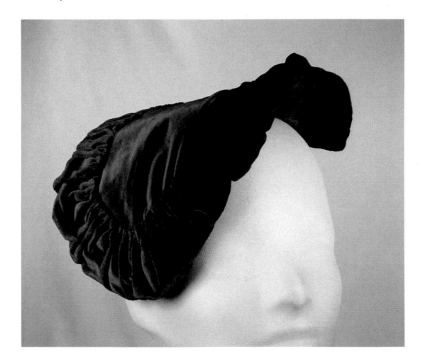

1940s green silk velvet with ruching around edges.

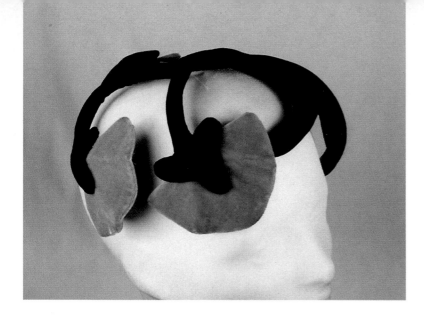

1940s black and pale blue "sculptural" hat; labeled Hattie Carnegie Original.

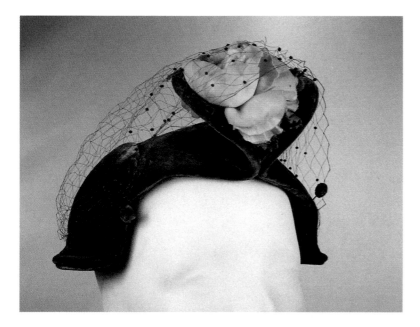

1940s rust brown velvet with chenille dotted veil and stand up floral; labeled Pauline Herman, Walnut at Nineteenth St., Philadelphia, Pa.

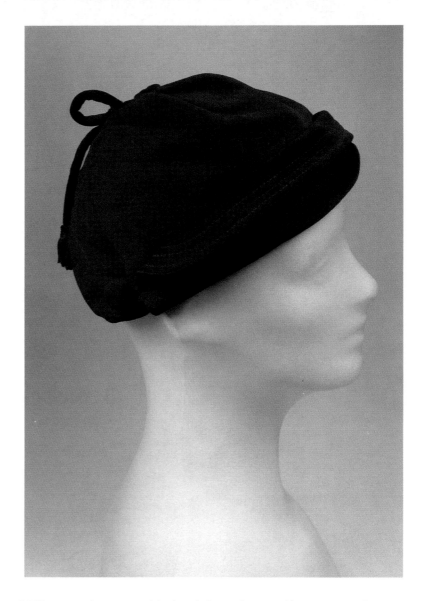

1950s rust velvet cap, with visor brim and covered buttons at sides, bow on top.

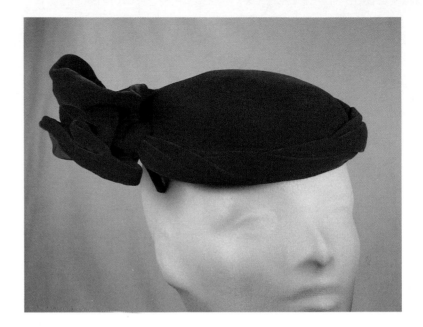

1950s red velvet "clip" hat with a "rolled velvet" edge and "knot-like" side decoration; labeled R.H. Stearns Co., Boston.

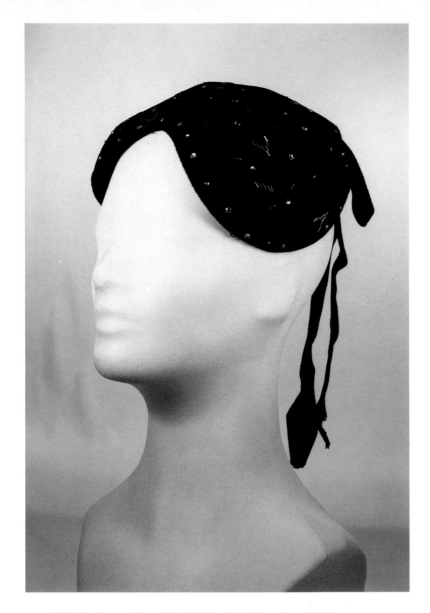

1950s black velvet, trimmed with clear bugle beads and rhinestones; labeled Reproduction of Legroux Soer, Paris.

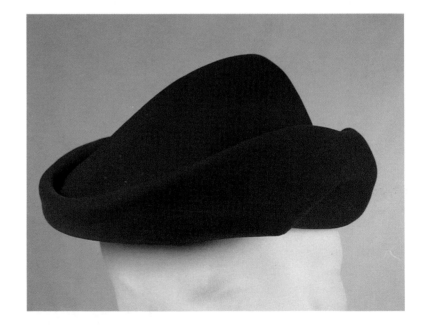

1950s red sculptured velvet; labeled Trébor Original, Hess Brothers.

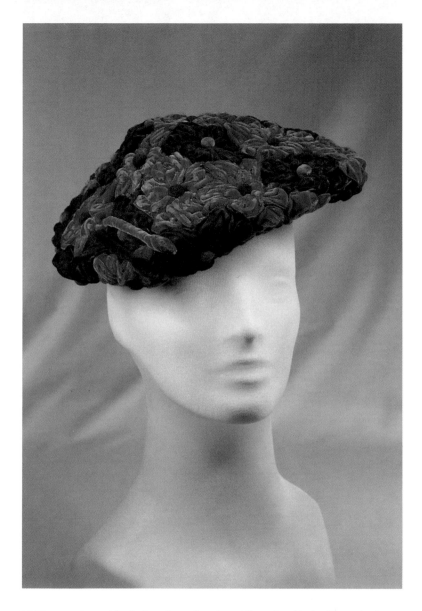

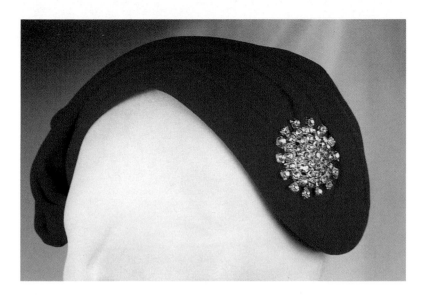

1950s red gathered velveteen with rhinestone decoration; labeled John B. Stetson, Fifth Avenue.

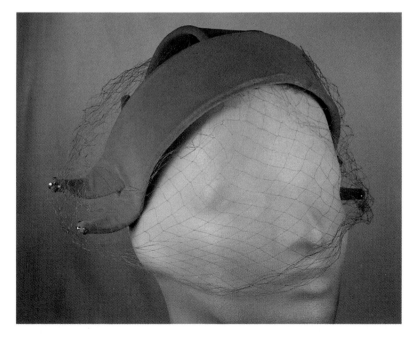

1950s purple and fuchsia velvet, floral motif made of tube-like velvet ribbon; labeled The Blum Store, Braagaard, Inc., New York. *Courtesy of Drexel Historic Costume Collection, Nesbit College of Design Arts, Drexel University.*

1950s "clip" hat in pale pink velvet, decorated with rhinestones and a pink veil.

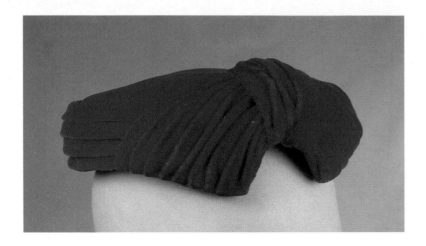

1950s orange velveteen cocktail hat; labeled Stetson, 1224 Chestnut Street, Philadelphia.

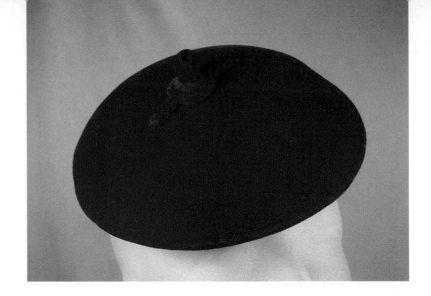

1950s red velvet clip on style hat, lined with printed silk which is dotted with rhinestones; labeled Saks Fifth Avenue, Millinery Salon.

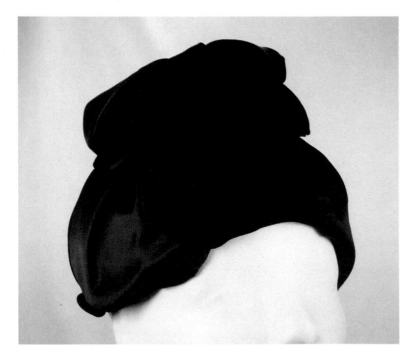

1950s black rayon satin and velvet with a dramatic high crown; labeled Don Anderson, New York.

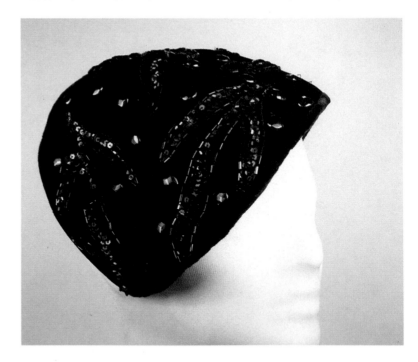

1950s black velvet, decorated with blue sequins and beads; labeled Dorothy Lovell Ltd. Original, Baltimore.

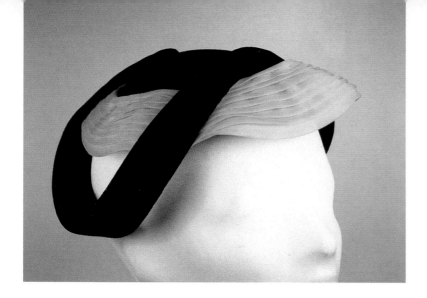

1950s black silk velvet with pink silk chiffon; labeled Solange de Fabry.

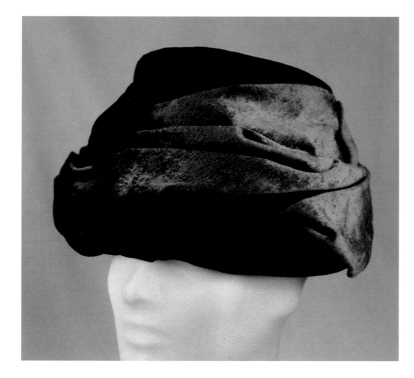

1950s black and gray silk velvet; labeled Anna, Astor Shop, Harrisburg, Pa.

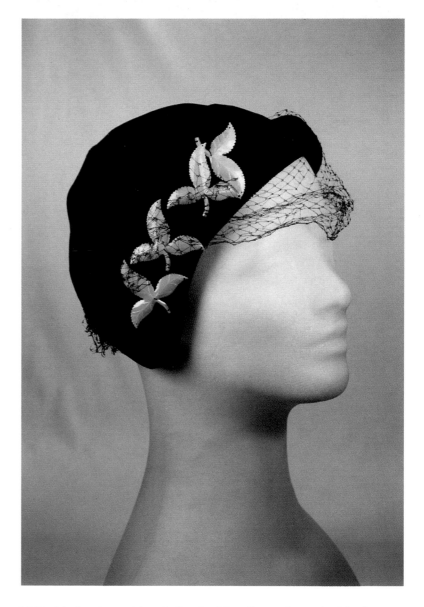

1950s black velvet with veil, lined with taffeta, trimmed with abalone shell leaves.

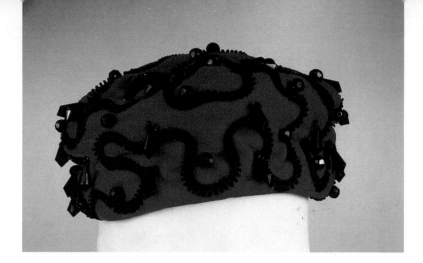

1960s pillbox of red velvet, decorated with black glass beads and appliquéd in black cord; labeled Brandt, New York.

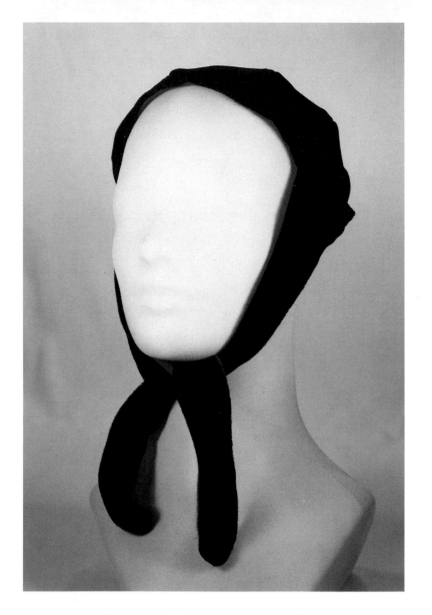

1950s red wool jersey and navy velvet reversible scull cap with chin tie.

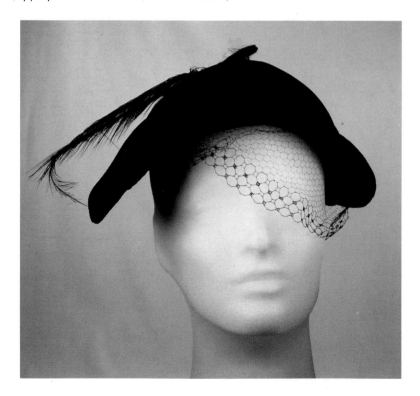

1950s black velvet hat, trimmed with a single feather; veil has two sizes of mesh, which is very unusual.

Mr. John

Mr. John's full name was John Piocelle. Before World War II, Mr. John was in partnership with Frederic Hirst in a business known as John Frederics. In the 1950s, he set up shop under his own name on West 57th Street in New York City. Reva Ostrow, New York accessories' designer, who has worked in the fashion industry for over twenty-five years, told me that "John was the designer," which is another way of saying the early John Frederics hats and the post-war Mr. John hats are the most exciting!

Mr. John reigned for many years from his white and gold salon. Each time he launched a new collection he published *Mr. John's Fashion News*. His models for these publications were often well-known socialites and movie stars. Mr. John died in 1993, the same year that the Philadelphia Museum of Art opened the inspirational exhibition, *Ahead of Fashion: Hats of the 20th Century*, from August 21 to November 7, 1993, organized by Dilys Blum. The *Bulletin* for the exhibition was dedicated to Mr. John.

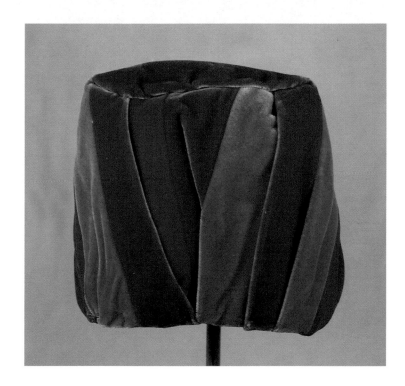

1950s "princess style" cap in shades of red and rose velvet, beautifully pleated; labeled Mr. John, Sydney of Albert.

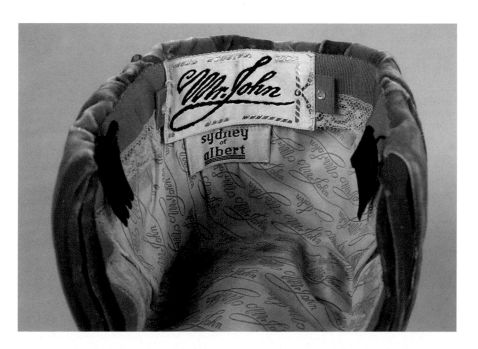

1950s Mr. John label and lining of "princess style" cap.

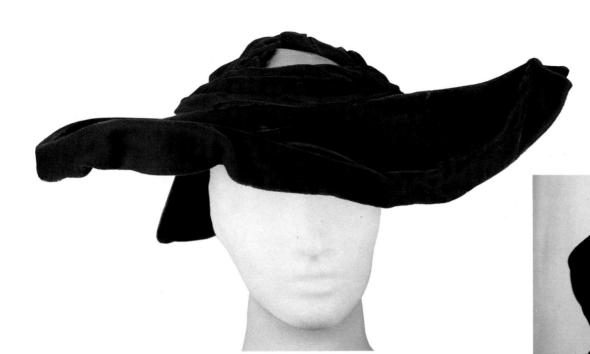

1950s open-crown burgundy rayon velvet, wide-brim wired for dramatic effect; labeled L. Bamberger & Co., Newark.

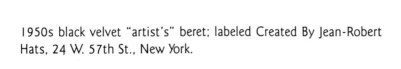

1950s black velvet "artist's" beret; labeled Created By Jean-Robert Hats, 24 W. 57th St., New York.

Not Exactly...

Inspiration for millinery does not always find expression in traditional materials. The milliner may conceive of a design for a hat that consists of an asymmetrical wire frame, decide to wrap the frame with metallic thread, and then add the finishing touch, a single, silk velvet rose.

For a period of time, a particular fabric, such as wool jersey, may become popular for millinery and then fade from popularity, leaving a small, difficult to categorize, group of hats behind. The genius of the milliner is not confined!

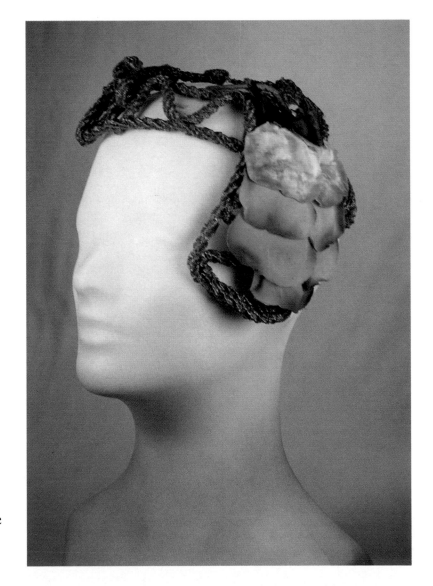

1950s wire frame covered with metallic braid, decorated with a single peach silk and velvet floral with green leaves.

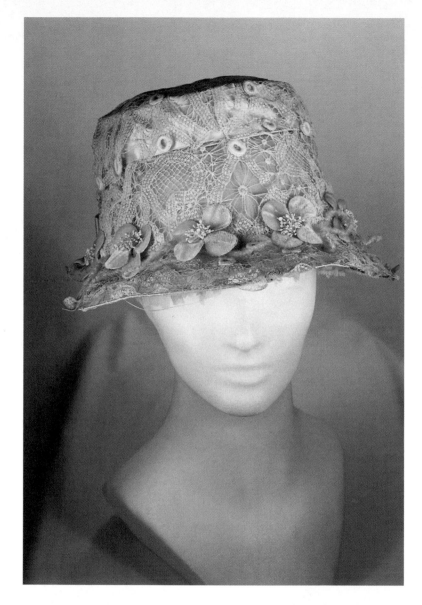

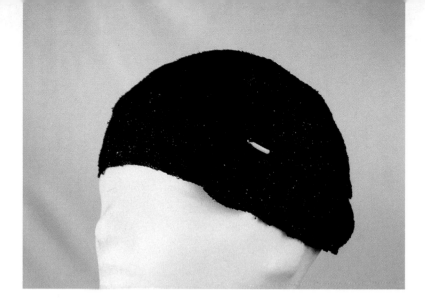

1920s black metallic knit cloche, decorated with a bow and a small bakelite ring, silk lined.

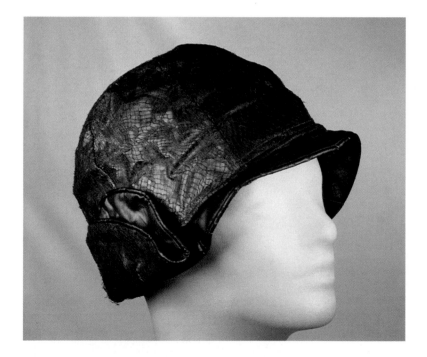

Ca. 1880 handmade lace over silk on wire frame, decorated with silk velvet flowers, silk and tulle lined, for a bride. *Courtesy of Alison Bartholomew.*

1920s toque with lace over gold metallic oil cloth., lined with black silk.

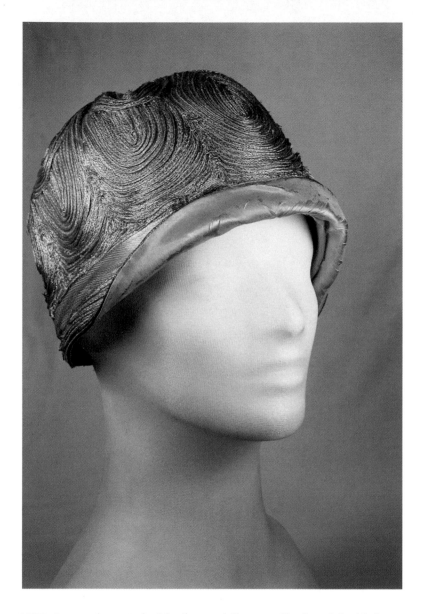

1920s toque, decorated with silver and lilac metallic thread, braided and applied in swirls, silk brimmed, taffeta lined. *Courtesy of Sharon Glosser.*

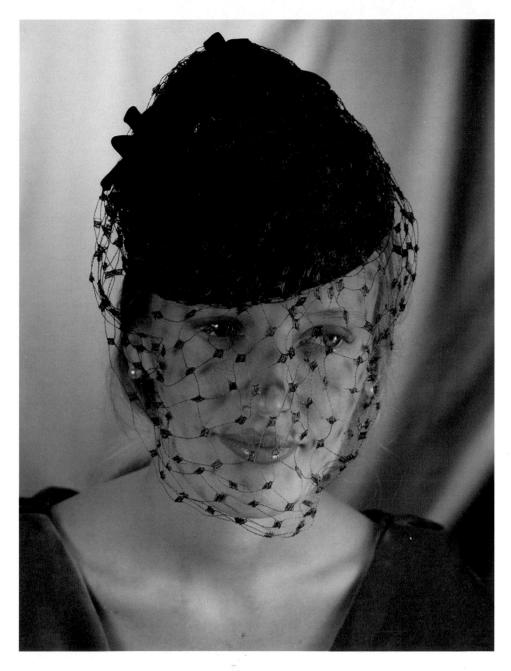

1930s "doll hat," very likely reissued in the 1960s, blue veiling wrapped around a pointed crown, satin bows all over; labeled Lilly's Dilly's, Designed by Lilly Daché. *Modeled by Marcie Behanna.*

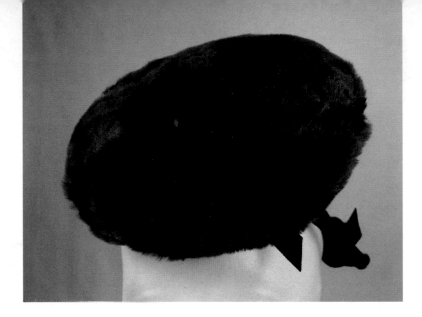

1930s Mouton lamb "doll hat" with brown felt strap; labeled New York Creations.

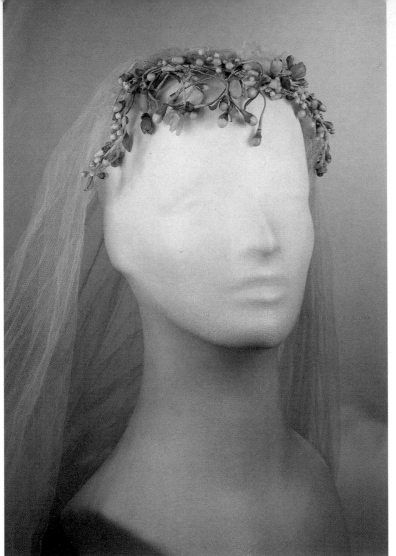

Ca. 1930 tulle veil with floral headpiece. *Courtesy of Alison Bartholomew.*

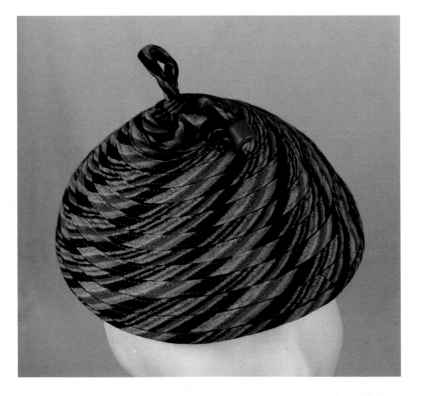

1930s wool jersey, sewn in strips in a circular fashion, gray, navy, green, and red multi; labeled Colby, Blum Store, Philadelphia.

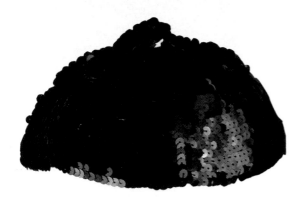

1940s black sequins on a net base.

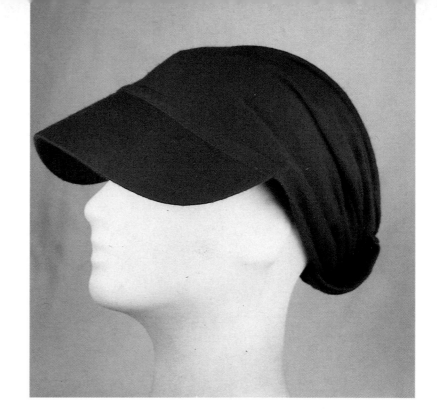

1940s rust colored wool jersey cap, with a visor, gathered in back.

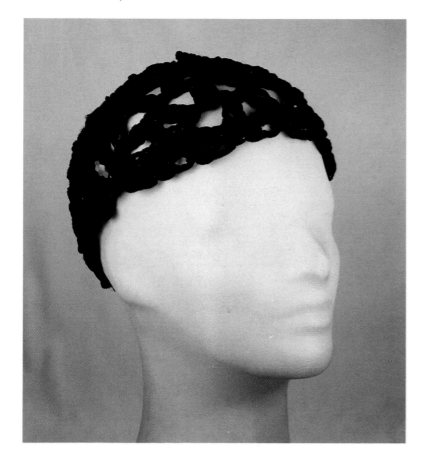

1940s black crocheted skull cap.

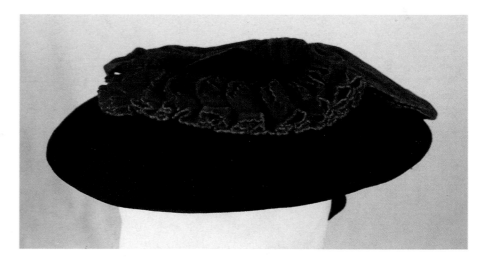

1940s black cord on a wire frame, trimmed with velveteen ribbon; labeled J.T. Schick & Son, 5240 Chestnut St., Philadelphia.

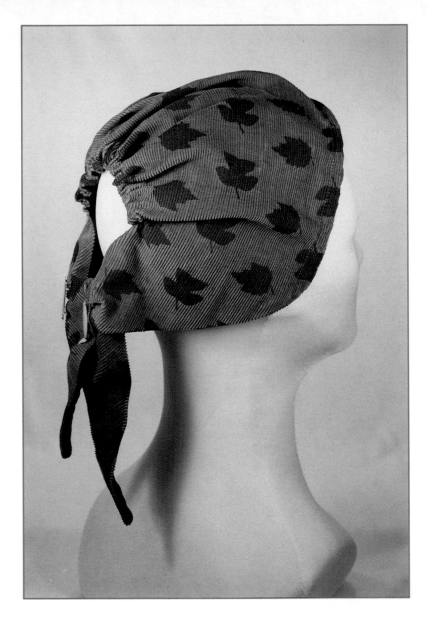

1950s green corduroy "clip hat," ties in back; labeled Vera.

Every woman consults her mirror and good sense in the arrangement of her hair... and in the choice of her hat.

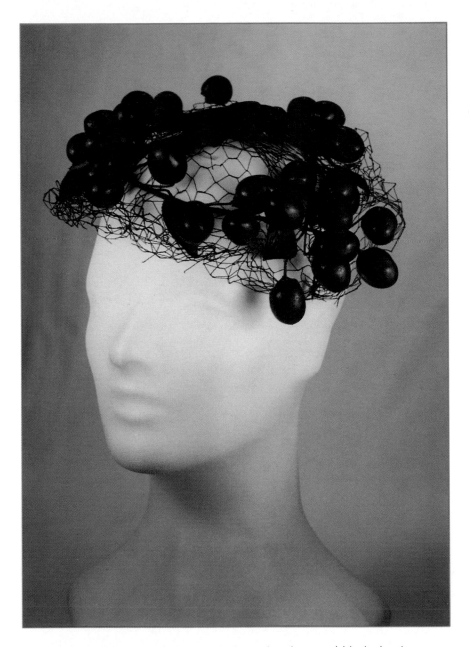

1950s black net hat, detailed with a velvet bow and black cherries and leaves. Fascinating.

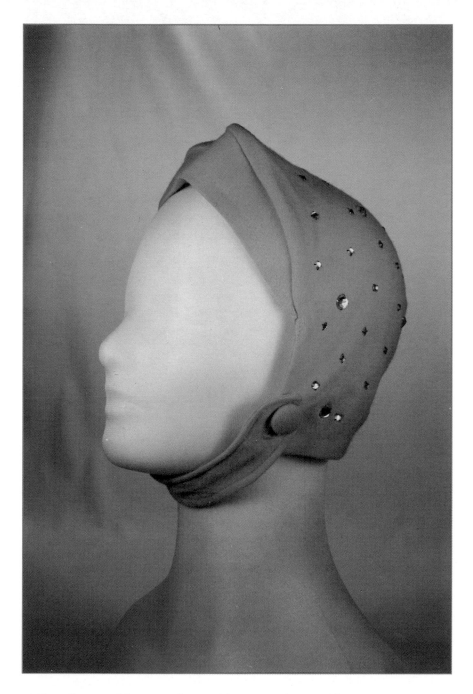

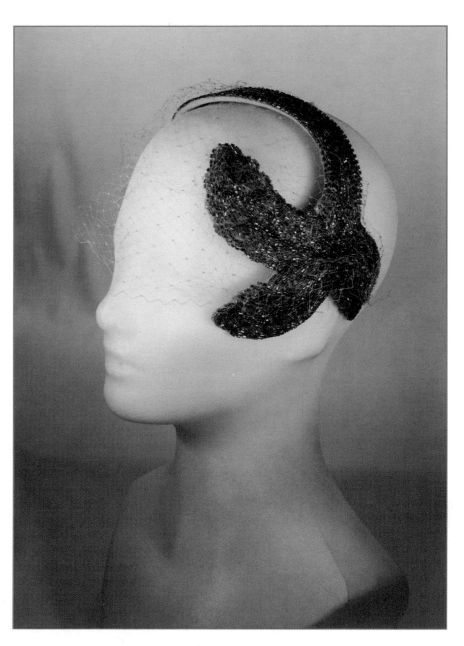

1950s yellow wool jersey scull cap with strap and covered buttons, studded with rhinestones, visor.

1950s blue silk clip hat with veil, entirely decorated with silver bugle beads.

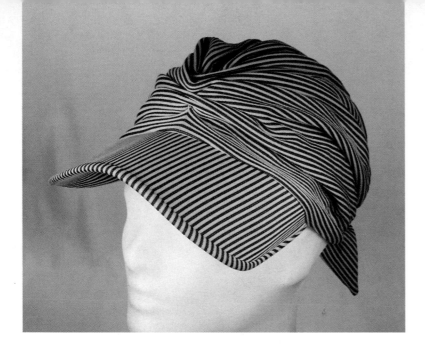

1950s brown and white rayon sports cap, possibly inspired by a railroad cap, large brim, knotted in back.

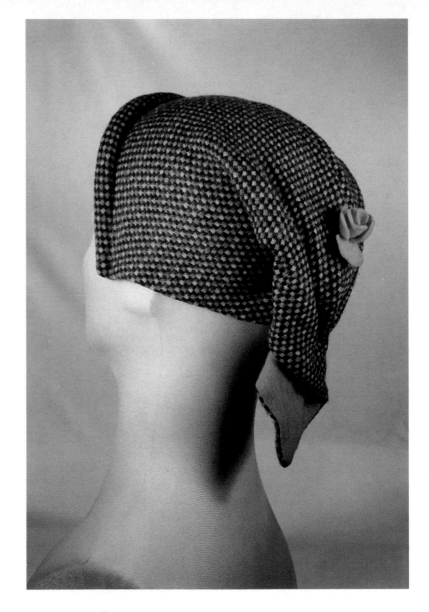

1950s gray, yellow, and white wool jersey clip, with a small yellow felt rose on the back. These hats hold great memories for me, as I wore them as a young girl.

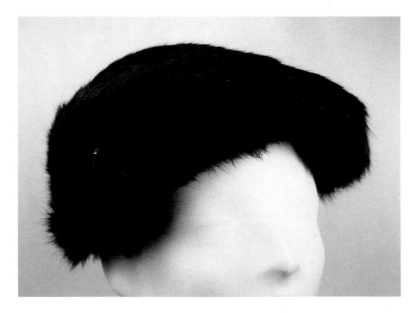

1950s fur, trimmed with a black satin bow and rhinestone clip; labeled Valerie Modes.

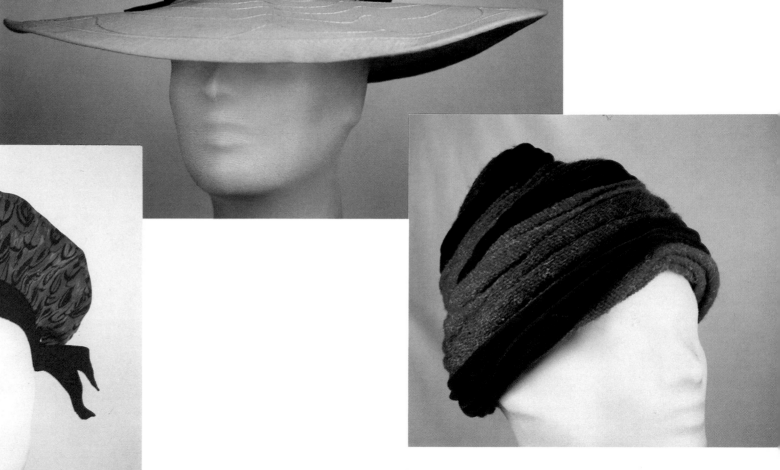

1950s linen picture hat, with a navy grosgrain ribbon band, trimmed with two covered buttons; brim is stitched in a series of decorative waves.

1960s turban style in shades of green and blue mohair with purple velvet; labeled Bamberger's, New Jersey.

1950s beret and matching scarf, made of very fine printed corduroy in shades of green, orange, and rust, with a black stretch brim; labeled by Vera.

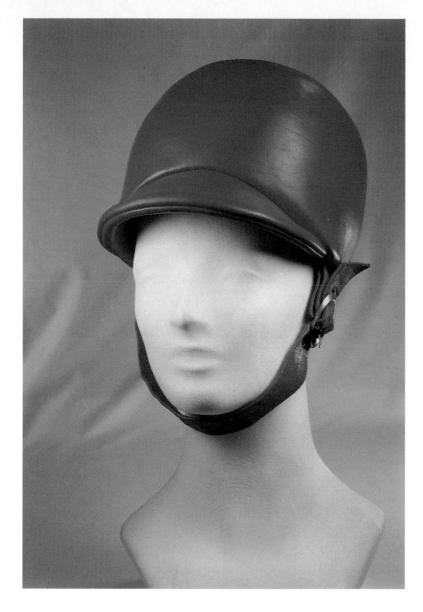

1960s red kid helmet with visor; labeled Emme, Inc., New York. *Courtesy of the Drexel Historic Costume Collection, Nesbitt College of Design Arts, Drexel University.*

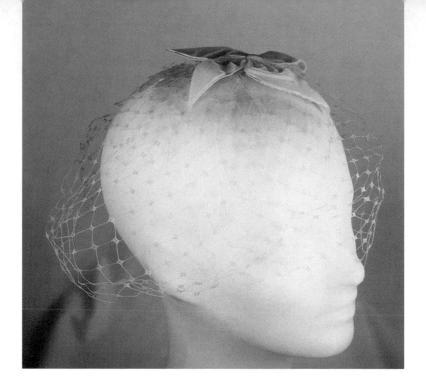

1960s "cage" hat of eggshell veiling with a silk bow on top.

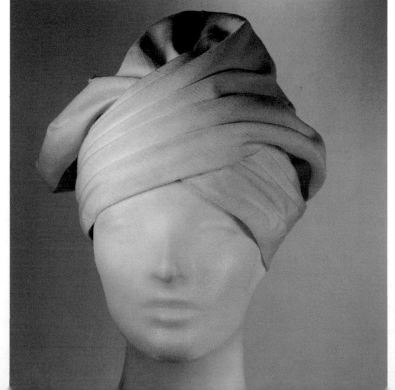

1960s white linen turban; labeled Mr. Martin.

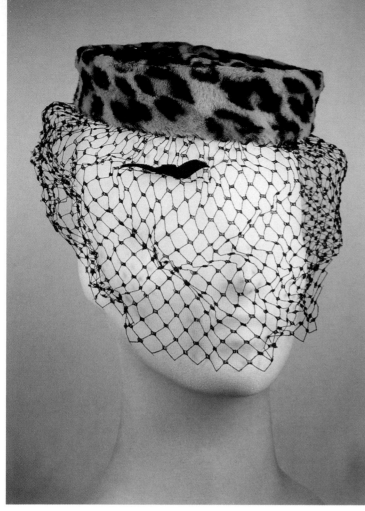

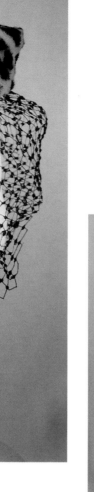

1960s "cage" hat with a velour leopard pillbox on top.

1930s wooden hat stand, painted and wearing its own hat!

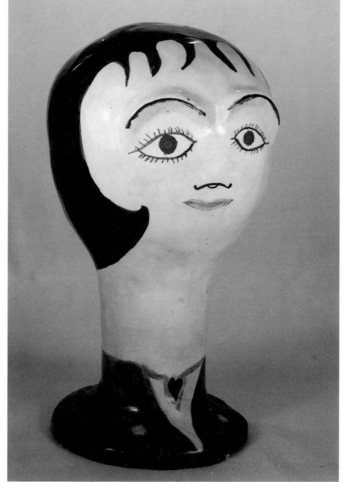

Ca. 1950s Stangl hat head, which originally had a wooden base. *Courtesy of Louise Stewart.*

❧ Flowers ❧

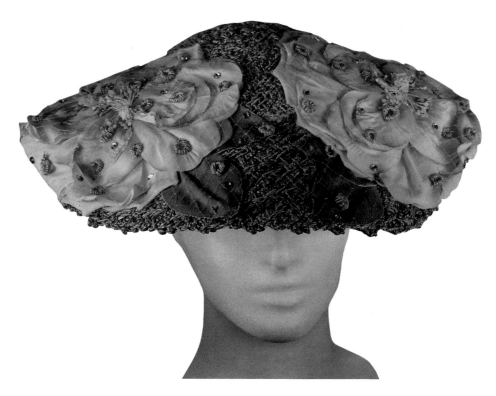

Milliners have been using artificial flowers since the mid-nineteenth century. Even earlier, dried, natural flowers may have been used to decorate bonnets. Cotton, feathers, silk, wax, and paper have all been used for making the add-on floral decorations. Horsehair, cord, and braid have been appliquéd or worked into floral patterns on hats. Felt has been used to make flowers, especially in the 1930s and 1940s.

Many of the flowers for millinery are imported, especially from France. Custom milliners usually learn the art of dyeing and curling silk flowers, and some even learn how to "ombre dye," which means dyeing flowers in related tones of monochromatic shading.

Flowers are a breath of spring in millinery, but it is not unusual to find a velvet or velour hat, which are traditionally winter or fall hat materials, decorated with flowers.

1940s natural straw, decorated with two large silk flowers, green leaves, rhinestones and net; labeled a Frances & Walter Nelkin hat.

1940s black straw "jockey" hat with a crown of cloth flowers; labeled French Room, T. Eaton Co., Limited.

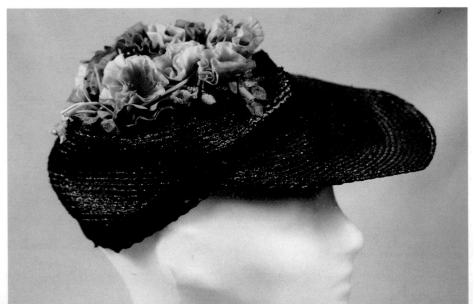

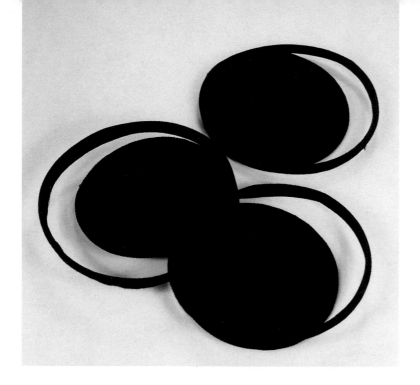

1940s black felt hat bodies, undecorated.

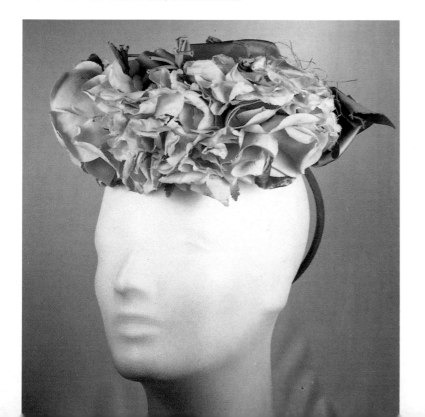

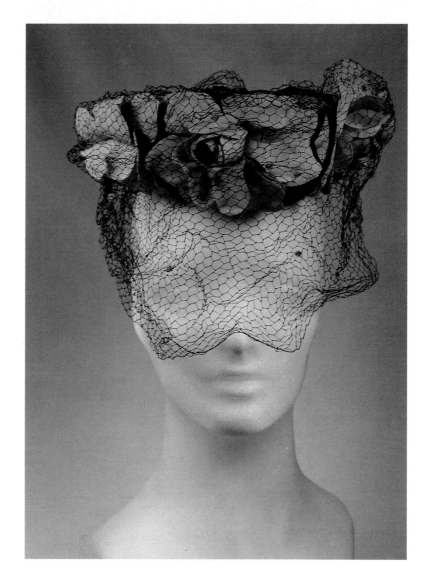

1940s beige fur felt, trimmed with cloth roses; labeled Marché Hats, New York.

1940s green silk satin with a profusion of pink and white cloth flowers.

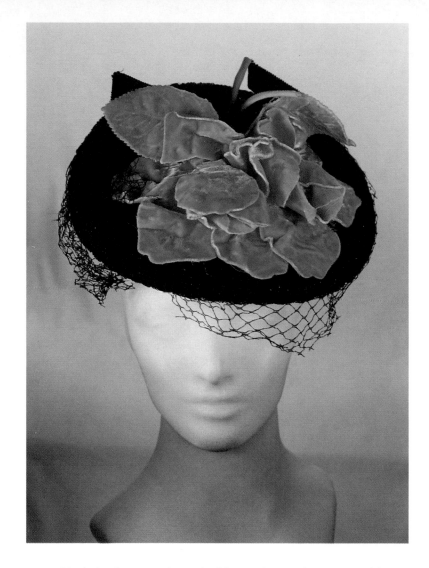

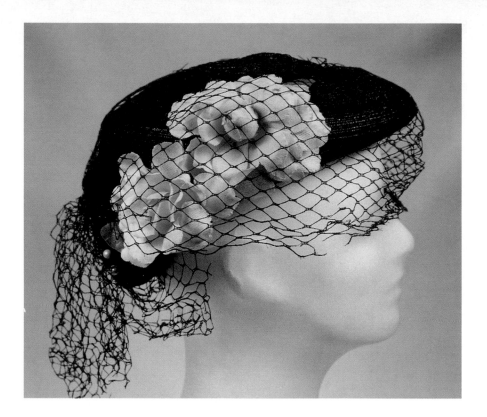

1940s navy straw, decorated with two large oyster white gardenias on each side, veil.

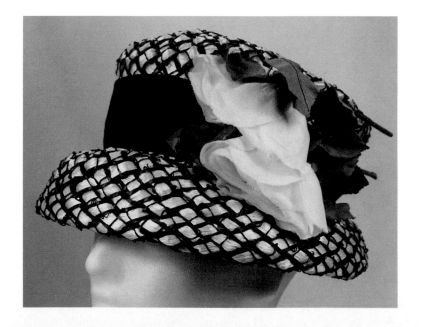

1940s black dyed straw, trimmed with two large velvet roses, with green cloth stems.

1950s black and white cellophane straw with a wide black velvet band and a large white silk rose; labeled Mr. Josephs, New York, H. Leh & Co., Allentown.

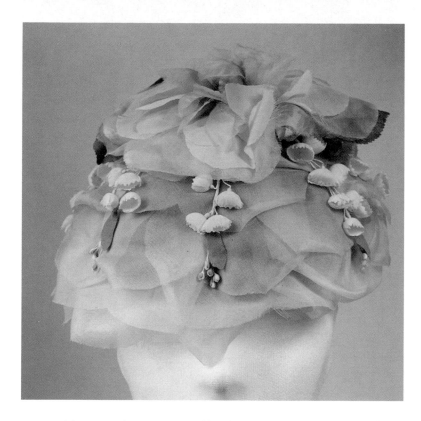

1950s white organdy over green silk, a large rose on crown, lilies of the valley cascading down from crown; labeled Gigi of New York.

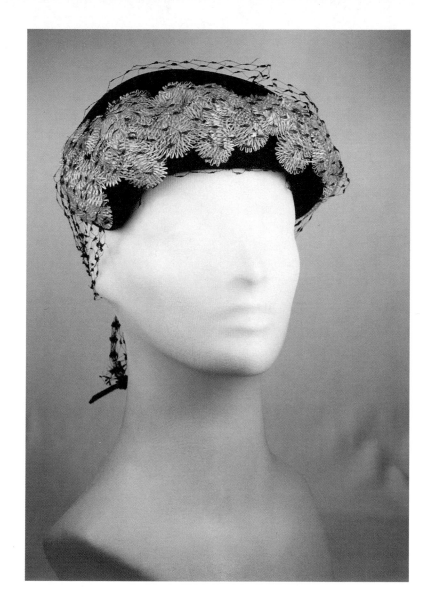

1950s pink horsehair florals on black velour base.

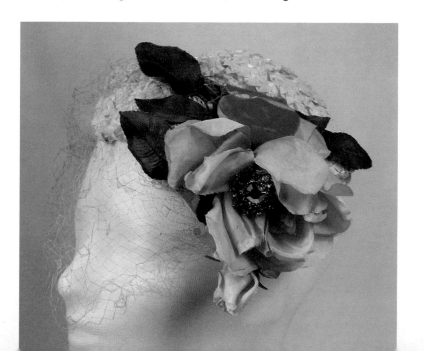

1950s white cellophane straw decorated with a large pink silk rose, with a rhinestone center; labeled Kurli-Kates, H. Leh & Co., Allentown.

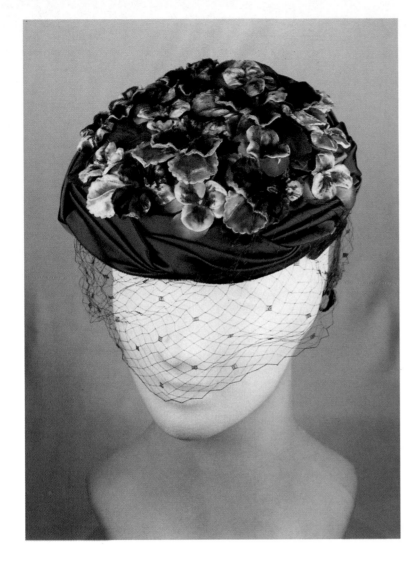

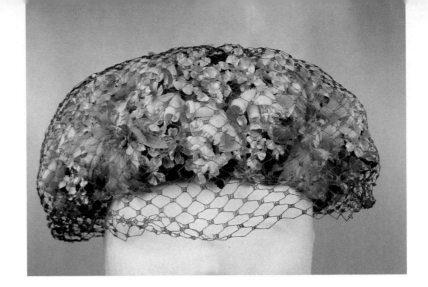

1950s miniature floral over net with all-over green veil; labeled Stetson, 1224 Chestnut Street, Phila.

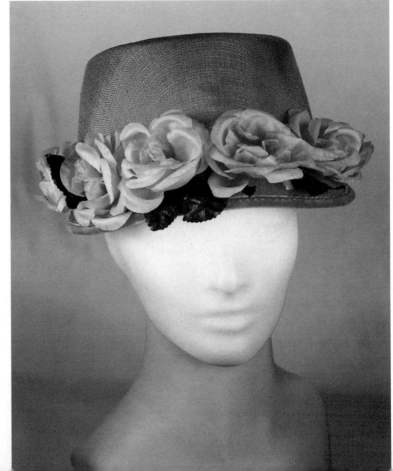

1950s purple satin hat covered with velvet artificial pansies and green silk leaves.

1950s pink rayon "hard hat" trimmed with pink rayon roses and green cloth leaves.

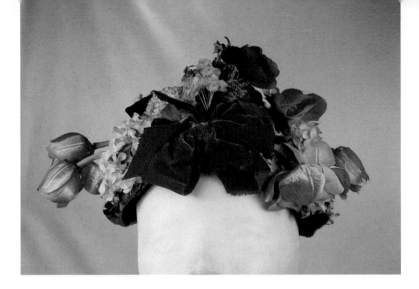

1950s floral, decorated with miniature flowers, velvet bows, green cloth leaves, and pink taffeta tulips; labeled Don Anderson, New York, Bonwit Teller.

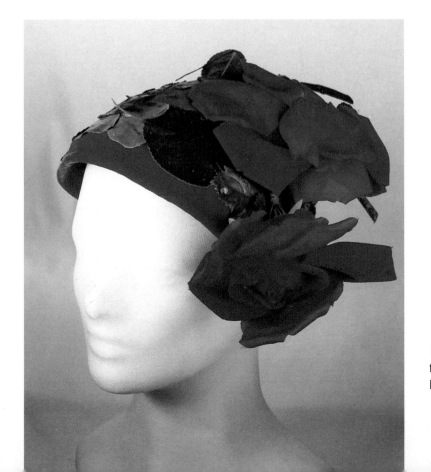

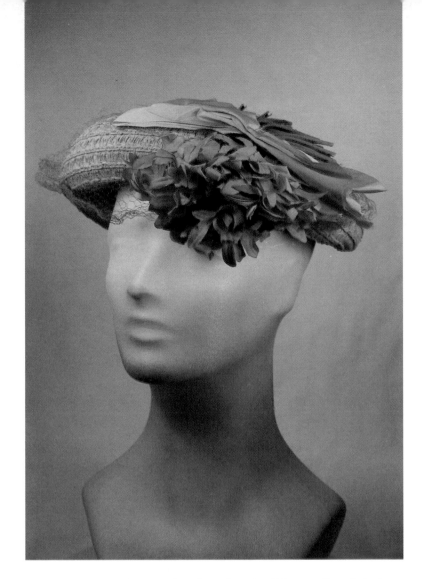

1950s pink straw, decorated with pink satin ribbon, veil and cloth flowers.

1950s red velvet over buckram, covered with green cotton leaves and trimmed with two large, red cloth roses; labeled Claire Hat Shop, Pottstown, Penna.

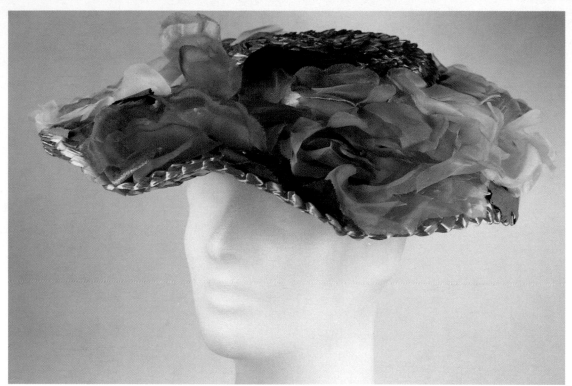

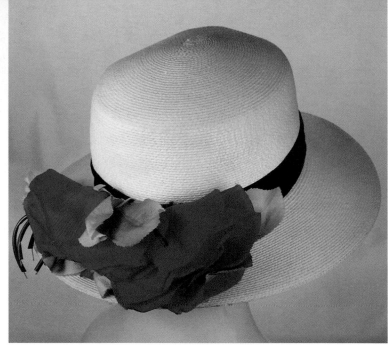

1950s white straw, with a black velvet band and silk flowers; labeled New York, Paris, Miss Gwenn Jr. Exclusive.

1950s rose cellophane straw, decorated with pink and white silk flowers, green paper leaves; labeled Evelyn Varon model.

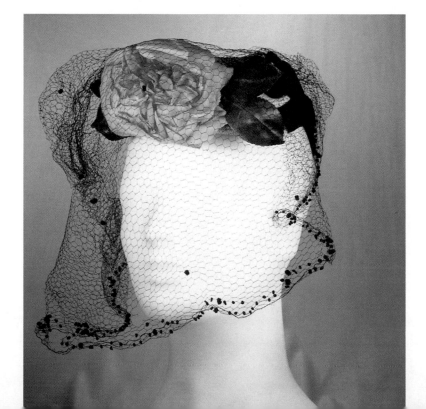

1950s pink silk floral with green cloth leaves, on wire frame, with chenille dotted veil; labeled An Original hatnip by Danciger.

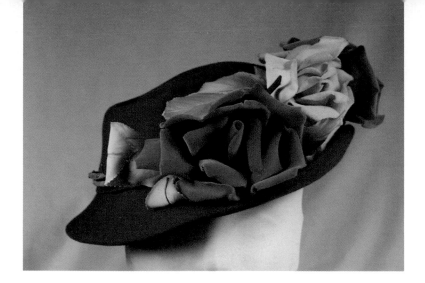

1950s burgundy velour trimmed with two large red and eggshell silk roses; labeled Chapeaux d'Art, 41 Coulter Avenue, Ardmore, Pa., *Courtesy of the Drexel Historic Costume Collection, Nesbitt College of Design Arts, Drexel University.*

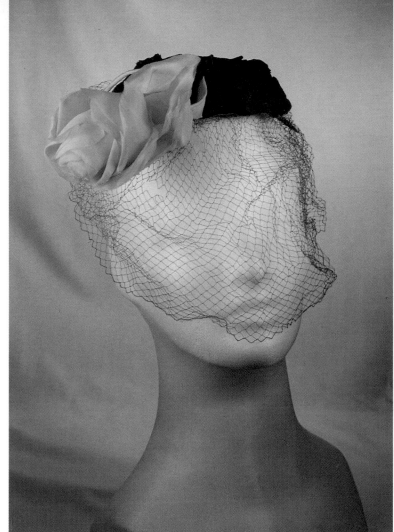

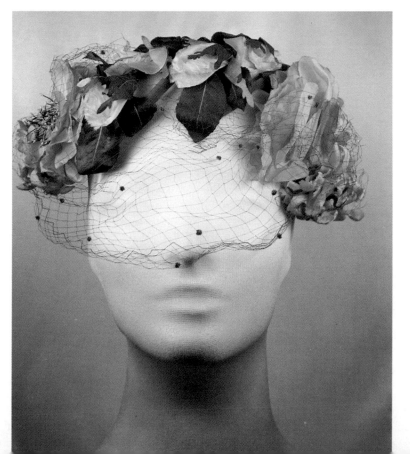

1960s "cage" hat with a small crown of artificial green leaves, trimmed with a single large yellow rose; labeled Miss Sally Victor, New York.

1950s floral on a velvet covered wire frame, chenille dotted veil; labeled Henri Bendel, New York.

❦ Contemporary Millinery ❧

My journey out of the past and into the millinery present took me into my own backyard, Philadelphia, where I found a microcosm of what is happening in the much larger, international millinery field.

At one time there were nineteen factories in Philadelphia that manufactured only hats, and countless custom milliners throughout the city. Hat labels suggest that there was a milliner on every block in the shopping districts of Philadelphia and New York. Small towns had speciality shops that boasted significant millinery business.

Hats went out of fashion in the 1960s, except for religious wear and weather protection. Only a small number of women continued to wear fashion hats. Within the last few years fashion hats have found their way back into all the major department stores, nestling among the winter caps, rain hats, and wide-brimmed, sun-protecting straws. Laura Ashley shops and other specialty shops are carrying impressive lines of very wearable, beautifully made hats. Models are shown wearing fashion hats on the runways and in fashion advertising, and fashion conscious women everywhere are putting hats back into their wardrobes.

In evaluating the state of contemporary millinery, it is valuable to look at design, manufacturing, and distribution. In doing this, I visited two programs at the college level that offer courses in millinery. There seems to be a growing custom millinery business, and there are some factories left that still make hats for women. I visited one such factory; the only one left in Philadelphia. Obviously, in order to market the hats, there must also be stores to sell them. In the past, there were many stores devoted exclusively to the sale of hats. Now, there are very few, but I visited one in an attempt to better understand the retail market for contemporary millinery.

Millinery at Drexel

Bella Veksler teaches fashion design, fashion history, and millinery at Nesbitt College of Design Arts, Drexel University. In addition to her teaching duties, she is curator of the Drexel Historic Costume Collection, an extensive collection of couture fashion and accessories dating from the early nineteenth century to the present.

A couture level seamstress who learned her skills in her native Russia, Ms. Veksler immigrated to the United States in 1974, first working as a fashion designer for Nan Duskin. She learned her millinery skills from her mother, an accomplished milliner in Russia, who had acquired her millinery skills in France.

Drexel offers the millinery course once a year for fashion design and fashion merchandising majors. Students must have a prerequisite accessories course, in which they learn such techniques as making silk flowers, textile dyeing, hand painting and embroidering silk, and beading. As Ms. Veksler points out, "every technique is beneficial for future milliners."

Drexel's millinery course includes all aspects of design, dyeing, shaping straw and felt, and trimming. As young designers, the students at Drexel are encouraged to relate each fashion accessory to the total appearance.

As a teacher of fashion, Ms. Veksler is a wealth of information. Discussing the future of millinery she believes that "femininity in fashion is gone," and that "everyone is like a maintenance man, carrying pocketbooks full of forgotten junk." She feels such large pocketbooks would be "unimaginable with a fancy hat." Although she loves millinery, she does not see a "big future " for the field.

Today, women do not learn the tradition of wearing hats from their mothers. Emphasis on hair styles, the informality of modern life, and a faster, business-like pace for women, have all contributed, Ms. Veksler believes, to the decline of millinery.

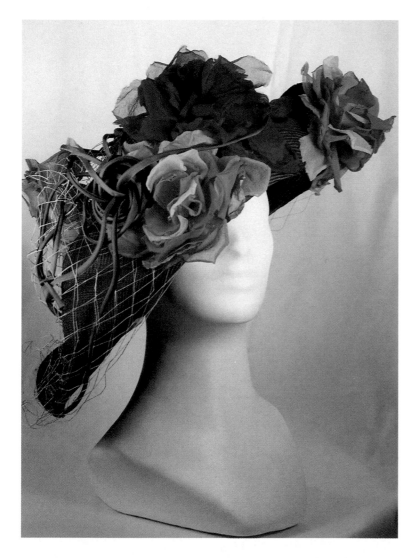

Contemporary mauve and purple "garden hat" made of dyed straw fabric, pure silk chiffon flowers, hand dyed with French dyes, thirty or more shades, stiff veil, green organza stems. Milliner: Bella Veksler.

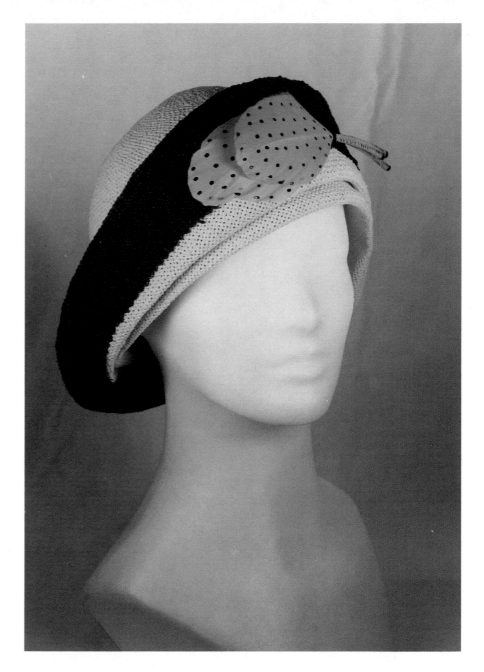

Contemporary pink and black dyed straw, based on free form draping on head block, flat pink feathers detailed with black dots. Milliner: Bella Veksler.

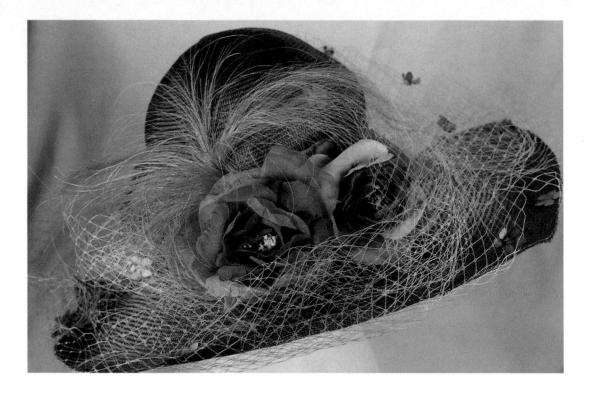

Contemporary lavender dyed straw, with handmade and dyed silk flowers. Feathers and veil are dyed to match petals of flowers. Hat designed to accessorize a lavender silk chiffon cocktail dress. Milliner: Bella Veksler.

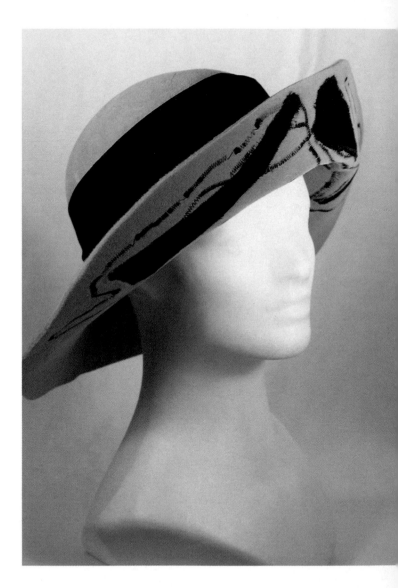

Contemporary brown velour, up-turned brim, net-covered crown, trimmed with pleated grosgrain silk ribbon. Milliner: Bella Veksler.

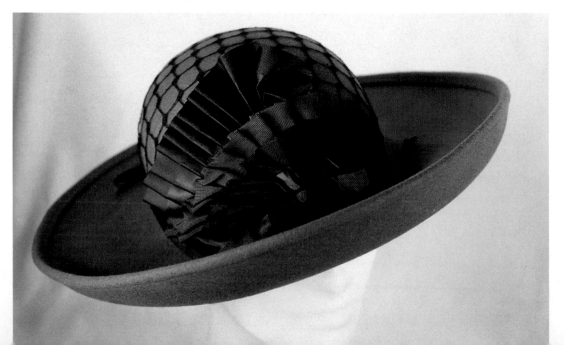

Contemporary beige, high quality, soft Italian velour, appliquéd in abstract designs in black pure silk velvet. Milliner: Bella Veksler.

Millinery at Moore

Alzie Jackson, Mr. Alzie, started making hats when he was sixteen years old. Now, more than fifty years later, he is still making hats, as well as teaching millinery in the Continuing Education Program at Moore College of Art.

Mr. Alzie, who has hats on exhibition at the Black Fashion Museum in Harlem and in the fashion collection of the Philadelphia Museum of Art, is an inspirational teacher. Many of his students live in the Philadelphia area, but one student mentioned that she had come "all the way from San Francisco to take the course."

When I visited the class, in preparation for photographing the students' work, I found the class so enjoyable that I stayed for two hours. At one point, Mr. Alzie was discussing his early millinery days in Harlem. He told the story of a large woman, chasing him with an umbrella, who was convinced that the hat she had purchased from him only a week before should not have come apart in the rain. "I told her I didn't make rain hats, but I knew then that I had better upgrade my materials."

Some of the students in Mr. Alzie's class are accomplished milliners, taking the class to brush up on their skills, or to learn new millinery techniques. Elizabeth Plepis, Mr. Alzie's assistant, is a designer at S & S Hat Company, in Philadelphia. A few students are new to millinery, but are obviously enthusiastic about every step in the process of making their first hats.

Mr. Alzie has said that there is "no front or back" to his designs, that his hats should be worn at "whatever angle is most flattering to the wearer."

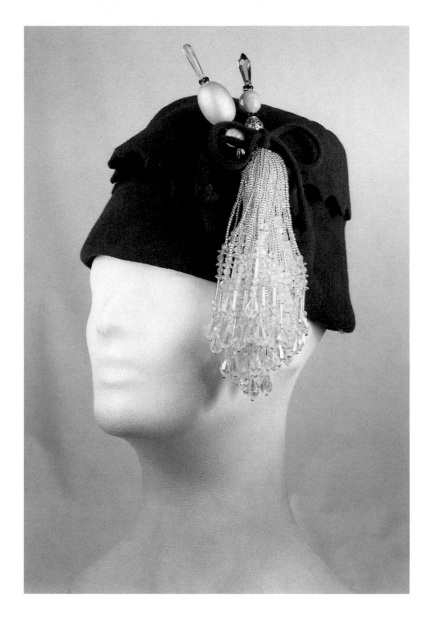

Contemporary green velour with stickpins and a beaded tassel, designed in multi-levels with a reversed-scalloped edge. A rounded felt bow completes a tailored, elegant look. Milliner: Mr. Alzie.

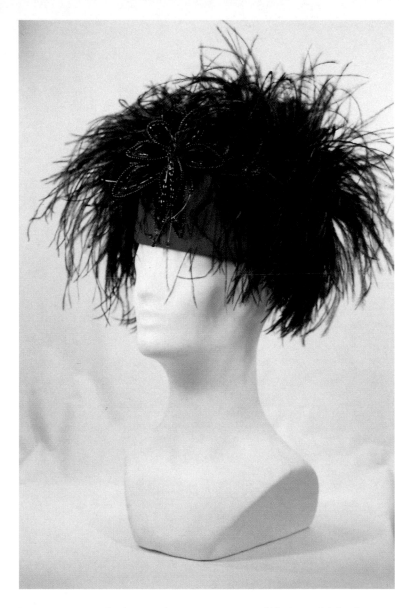

Contemporary red velour with an arrangement of black ostrich feathers and with a black jeweled ornament. Milliner: Mr. Alzie.

Contemporary purple velour skullcap, decorated with three rows of rhinestones, and large silk and velour flowers at each side, also rhinestone decorated; same color veil. Milliner: Mr. Alzie.

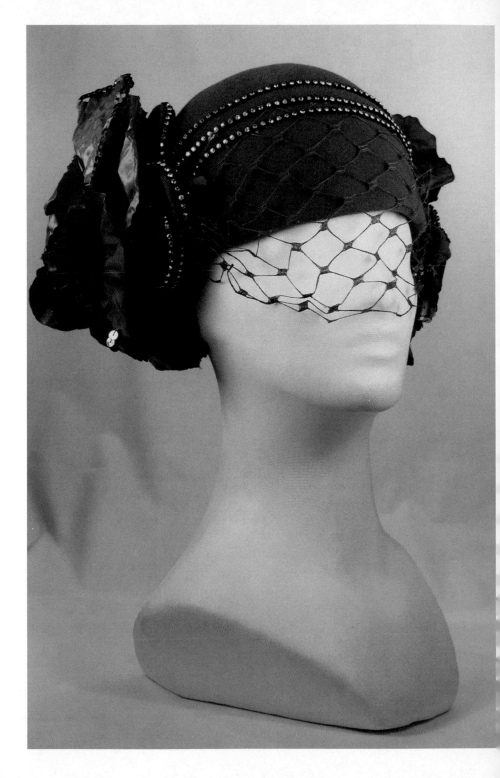

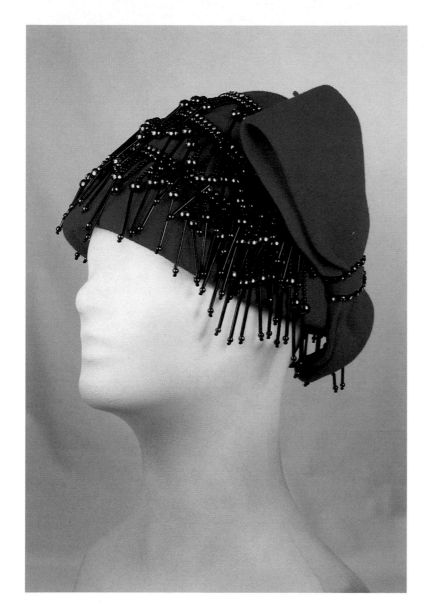

Contemporary red felt with an elaborate cascade of bugle beads in a contrasting color, and a large flat side bow, trimmed with beads. Milliner: Mr. Alzie.

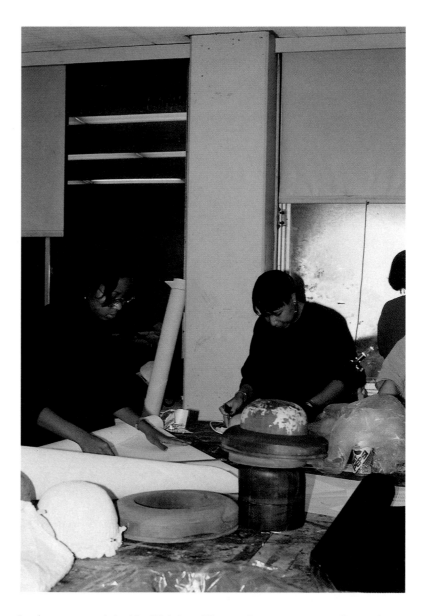

Students at work in Mr. Alzie's millinery class at Moore College of Art.

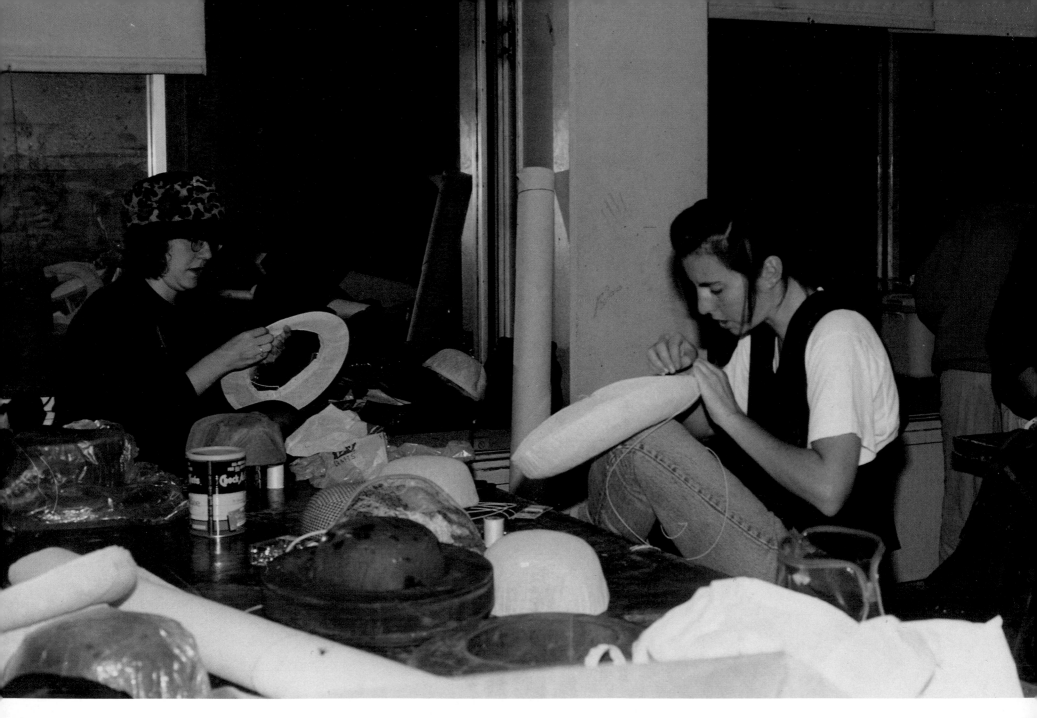

Students at Moore sewing buckram brims.

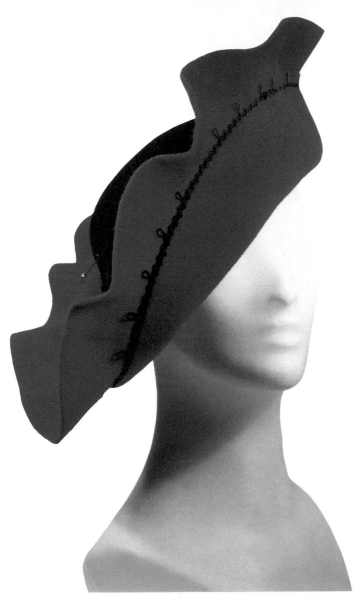

Contemporary red and black velour. "My first hat with Mr. Alzie in 1994." Milliner: Elizabeth A. Plepis, assistant to Mr. Alzie at Moore, a designer for S & S Hats.

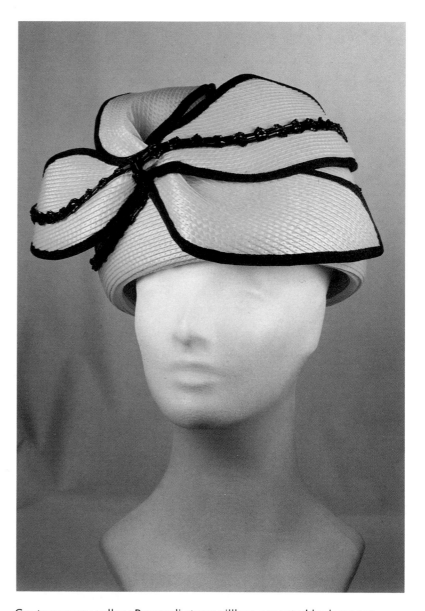

Contemporary yellow Romandi straw pillbox, accented by large petals, trimmed with black grosgrain and a black bugle bead and faceted button braid. Milliner: Elizabeth A. Plepis.

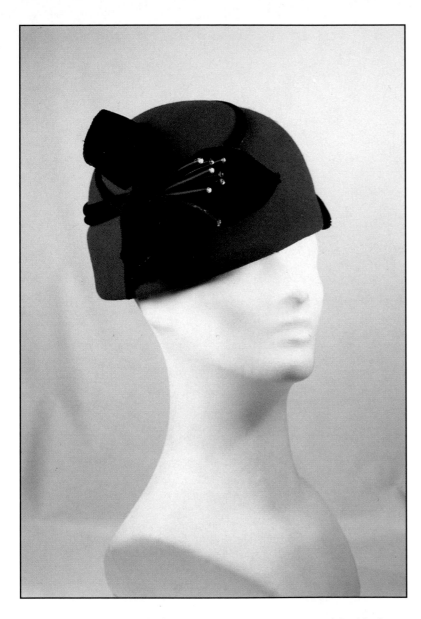

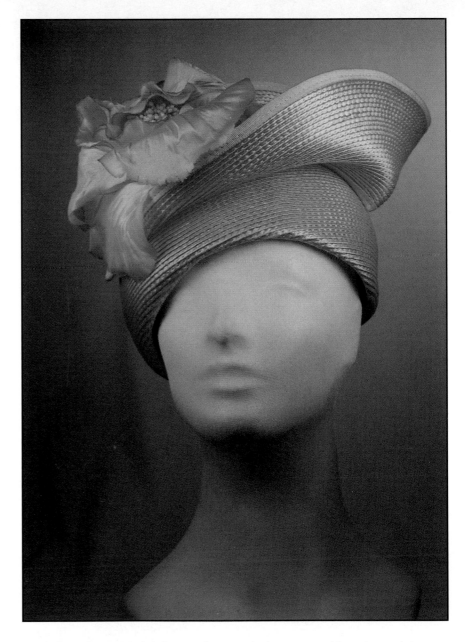

Contemporary burgundy felt in a spiral design, accented by black velvet cording, black velvet flower and rhinestones. Milliner: Elizabeth Plepis.

Contemporary pink Romandi straw cloche, accented by a large pink silk flower. Milliner: Elizabeth Plepis.

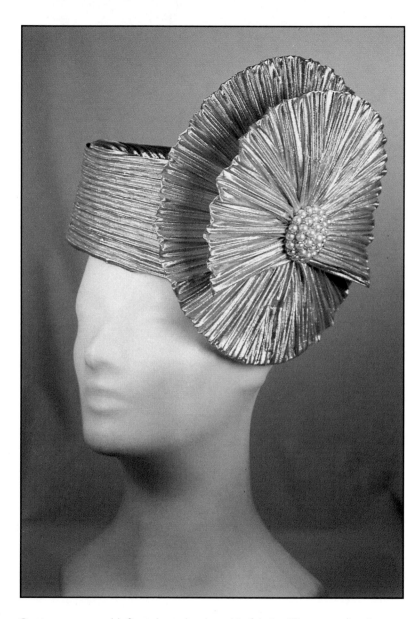

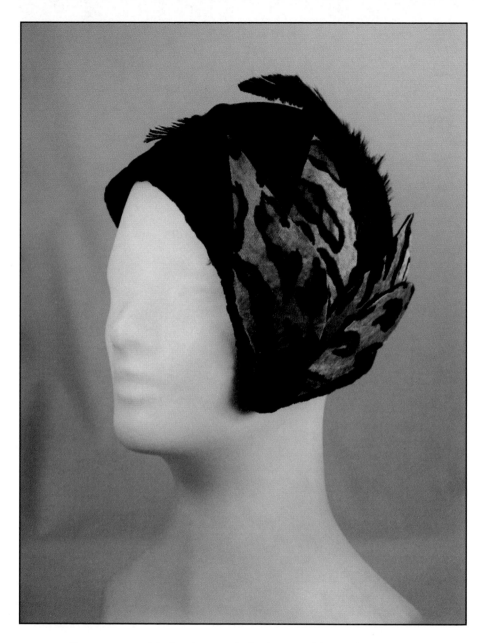

Contemporary gold, fine pleated onion skin fabric pillbox, on a buckram base, elaborate circular and semi-circular side decorations, artificial pearls at center. Milliner: Betty Pearson of Hatitudes.

Contemporary black velour with feathers and leopard accents over buckram frame. Milliner: Betty Pearson.

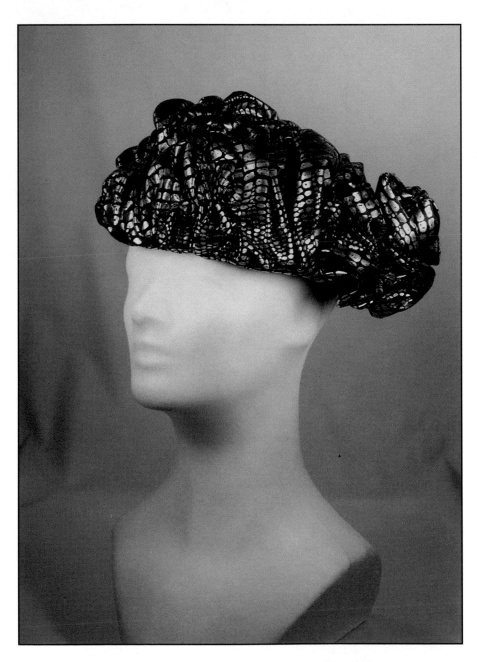

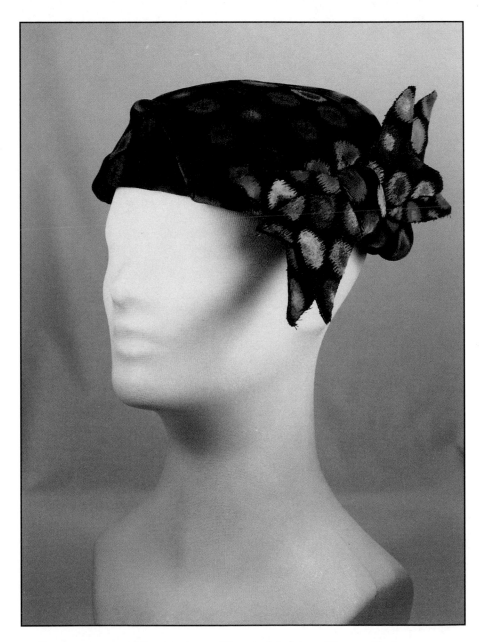

Contemporary iridescent green, lilac, and black lamé with a large rosette, over a buckram frame. Milliner: Lena Campbell.

Contemporary small velvet hat, with colorful dot motif, on a black background, and double bows on one side, "my first attempt at millinery." Milliner: Betty J. Rodgers

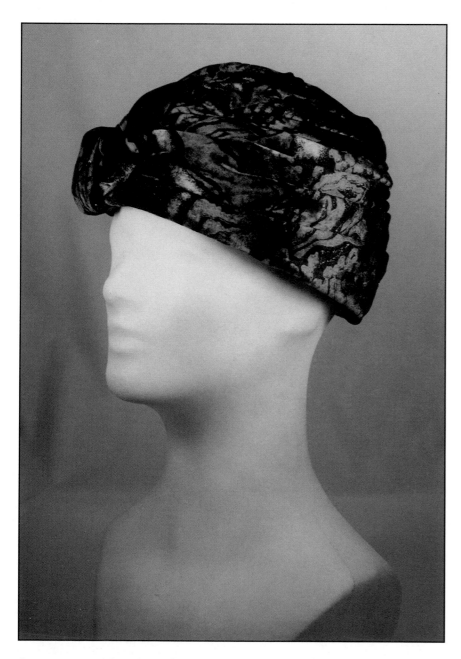

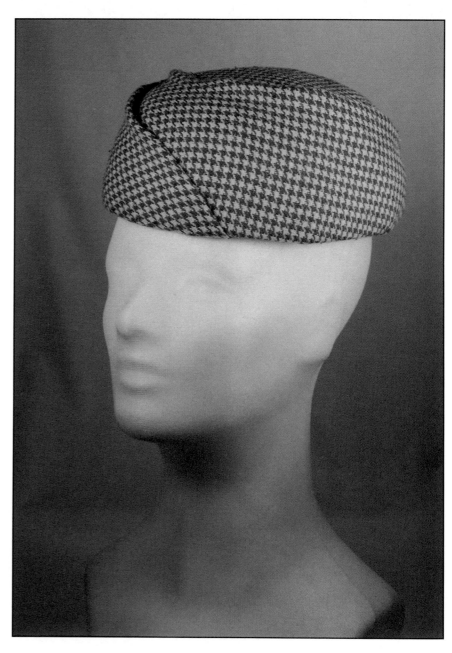

Contemporary multi-colored green, gold, and black velvet fabric draped on a buckram frame. Milliner: Girlee Gould.

Contemporary tan and brown houndstooth on buckram frame, "my first hat." Milliner: Helen Gonzalez.

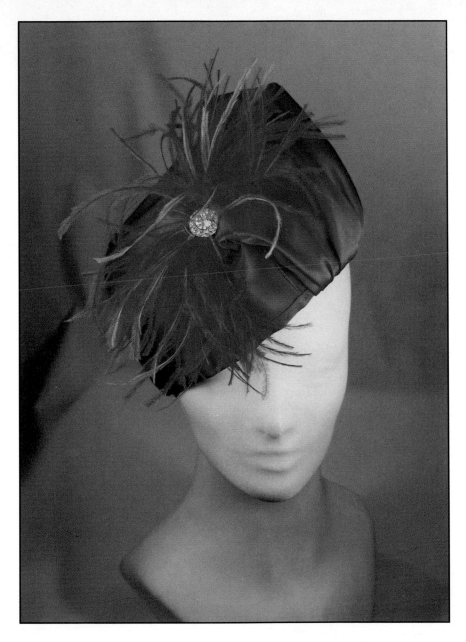

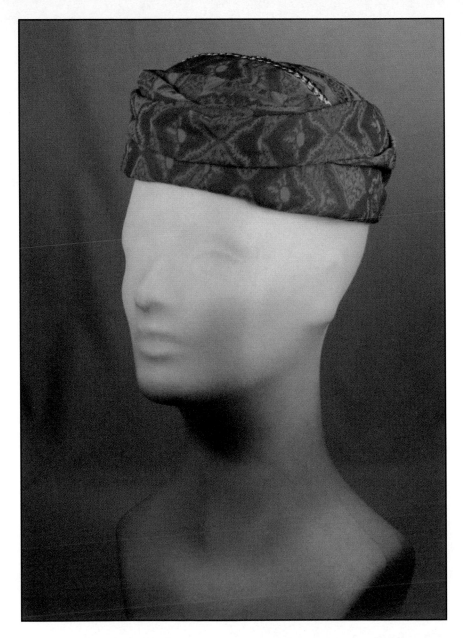

Contemporary bright pink antique satin, detailed with feathers and a rhinestone button, made on a buckram frame, "my first hat." Milliner: Margaret Fahringer.

Contemporary multi-colored jacquard, draped with gold braid across top, buckram foundation. Milliner: Monica Moore Boyer.

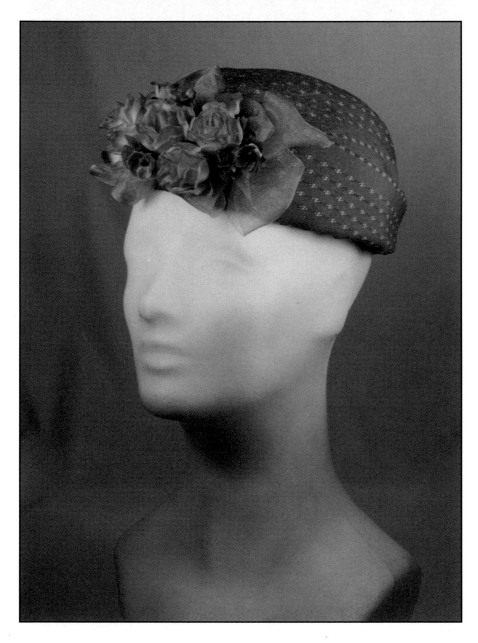

Contemporary little girl's hat, blue fabric with blue and pink flowers, draped on a buckram frame, "for my three year old niece." Milliner: Alice Dommert.

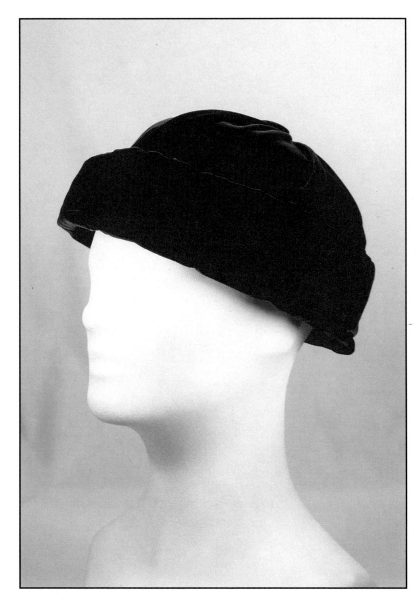

Contemporary chocolate brown rayon velvet with self button, "riding style," on a buckram frame, "my first hat." Milliner: Carolyn Rhodes.

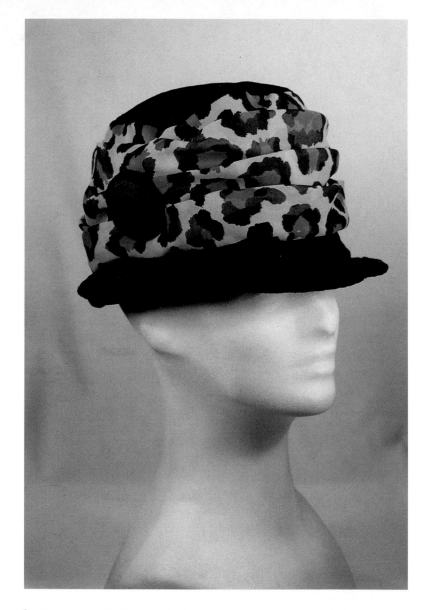

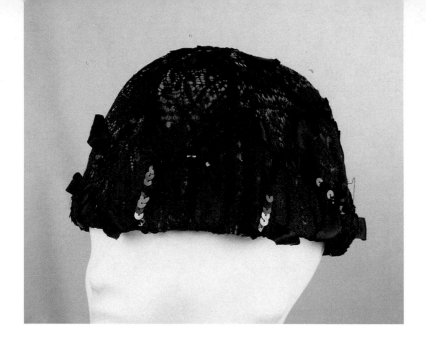

Contemporary turquoise knit velour, overlaid in black lace, satin ribbon, and black sequins on a buckram frame, reinforced with millinery wire to create facets, "my first hat." Milliner: Samuel Staten, Sr.

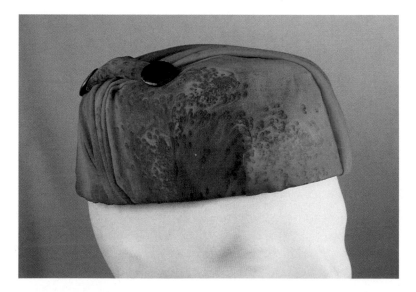

Contemporary black crushed velvet "scrunch style" cloche with multi-fold drapes of silk chiffon in a leopard print. Milliner: Ellen Gobler, Pure Presents.

Contemporary "tea hat" in turquoise silk chiffon with blue shell buttons on a buckram frame, "my first try at buckram framing." Milliner: Ellen Gobler, Pure Presents.

142

S & S Hat Company

A stone's throw from the new Philadelphia Convention Center, S & S Hat Company has been family owned and operated since 1923. Nestled among boxes of trimmings, bolts of material, and long rows of power machines, the designers have carved out their niches mostly close to the windows. On a clear day, you can see the rows of brick buildings catching the morning sun across the city. It's a stimulating, colorful place. Rows of hat trees, offering up the next season's designs, are lined up for inspection.

Jay Foreman, co-owner of the hat factory with his cousin, Mike Saft, introduced me to Alvin Foreman and Harry Saft, still active in the business. A floor to ceiling selection of wooden hat blocks speaks, more clearly than anything else, about the company's past. Mr. Foreman said that years back they were "throwing head blocks into fire barrels on 12th Street, never imagining that anyone would want last year's styles." Now he has a block re-made when it begins to show significant wear, in an attempt to preserve the past.

When I visited S & S, I had the rare opportunity of watching a blocker at work. The process of making a felt hat has not changed much since earliest times. The felt hood is soaked overnight. The blocker begins work early in the morning, stretching the wet felt over wooden hat blocks, a very strenuous job. The hat is then "seamed" with hot steam, and placed in a "hot box" to dry. The blocker must be agile, highly skilled, and very strong!

Don Andersen, Bellini, Brenda Waiters Bolling, and Tim Crawford, all top millinery designers, work for S & S. I was impressed with the diversity of styles the company offers, and my behind-the-scenes tour gave me new respect for the millinery field.

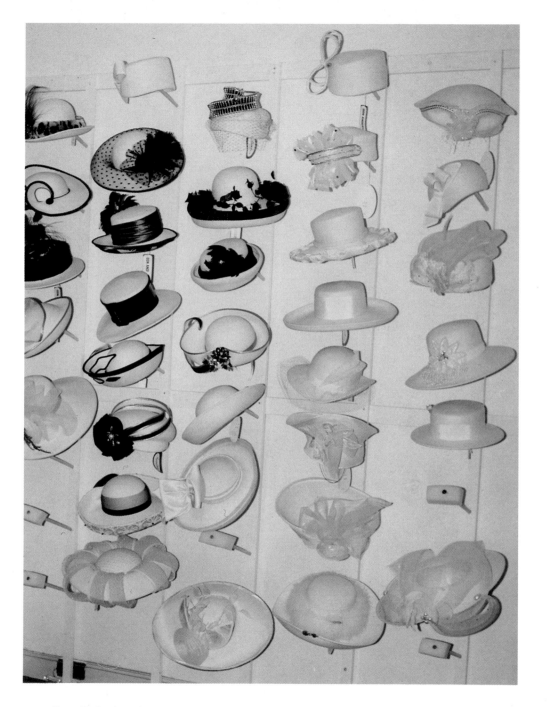

A wall of white hats at S & S Hat Company in Philadelphia.

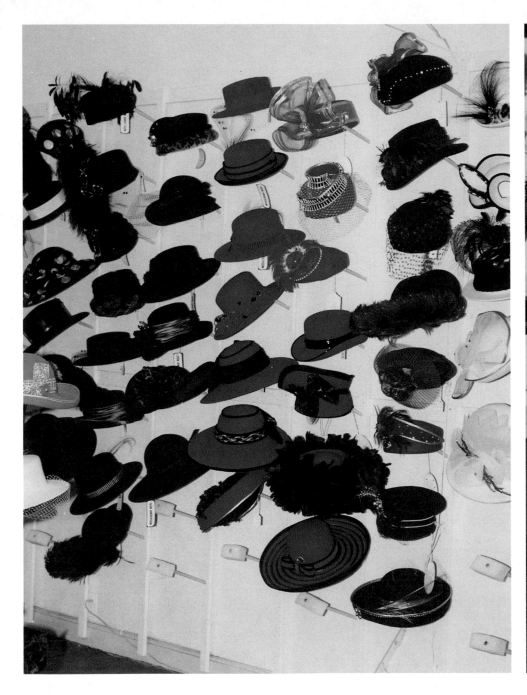

Colorful felts and velours.

Colorful soft velvets.

144

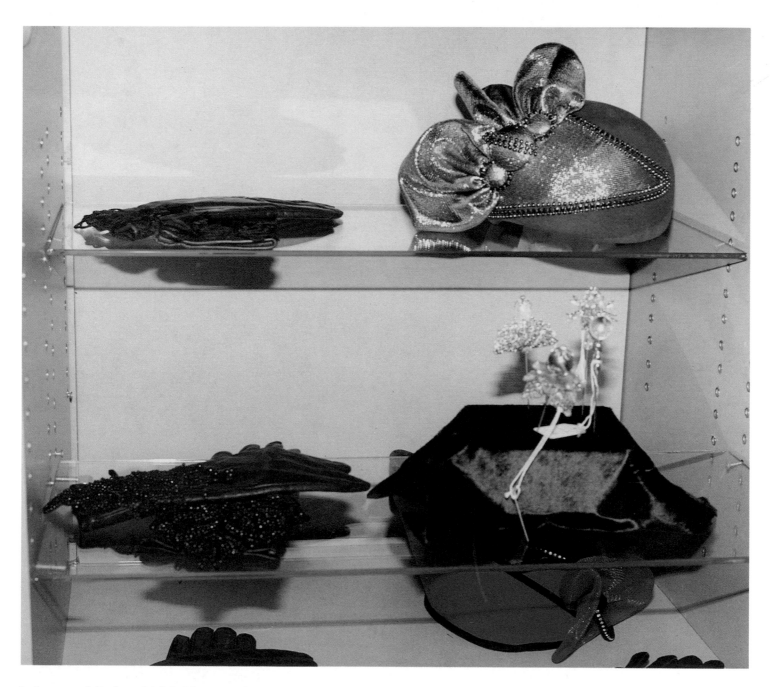

A showcase full of special S & S hats.

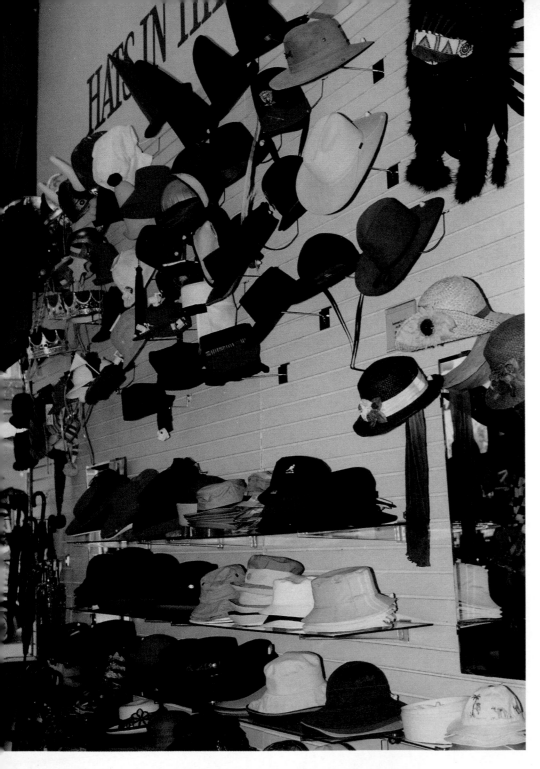

Hats In The Belfry

Tabytha Campbell presides at *Hats In The Belfry* at 3rd and South Streets in Philadelphia. The "incredible hat shop," as it's called, has five company-owned stores. The first store opened in Annapolis, Maryland, fourteen years ago. The shop carries a diverse line of hats for men and women. Designers Erik Javits, Steven Kokin, Helen Kaminski (Australian), and Don Anderson are favorites with customers. Ms. Campbell sees a trend toward big hats for women. When a movie is released, such as *Four Weddings and a Funeral*, portraying the ambiance of millinery, this stimulates buying. Buyers are still coming to the store to buy the Stetson that Harrison Ford wore in the movie, *Indiana Jones and The Temple of Doom*.

Although the shop sells a lot of baseball caps, especially by Kangol, it sells lots of western hats by Stetson, and driving hats. Women tend to buy for special occasions, especially weddings.

A number of women bought wide-brimmed straws to wear to the Kentucky Derby. Sports related hats are always of interest, and many avid skiers are choosing an unconventional look for the slopes, especially the large "Mad Hatter" top hats.

A wall of hats at *Hats In The Belfry* in Philadelphia.

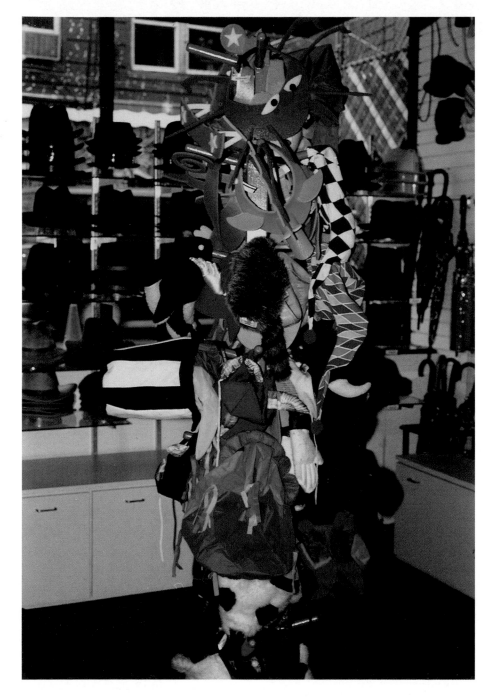

Fun hats.

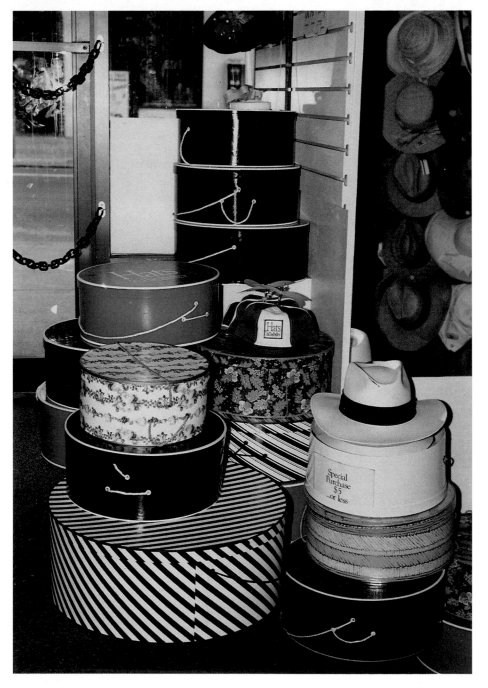

Hatboxes are popular.

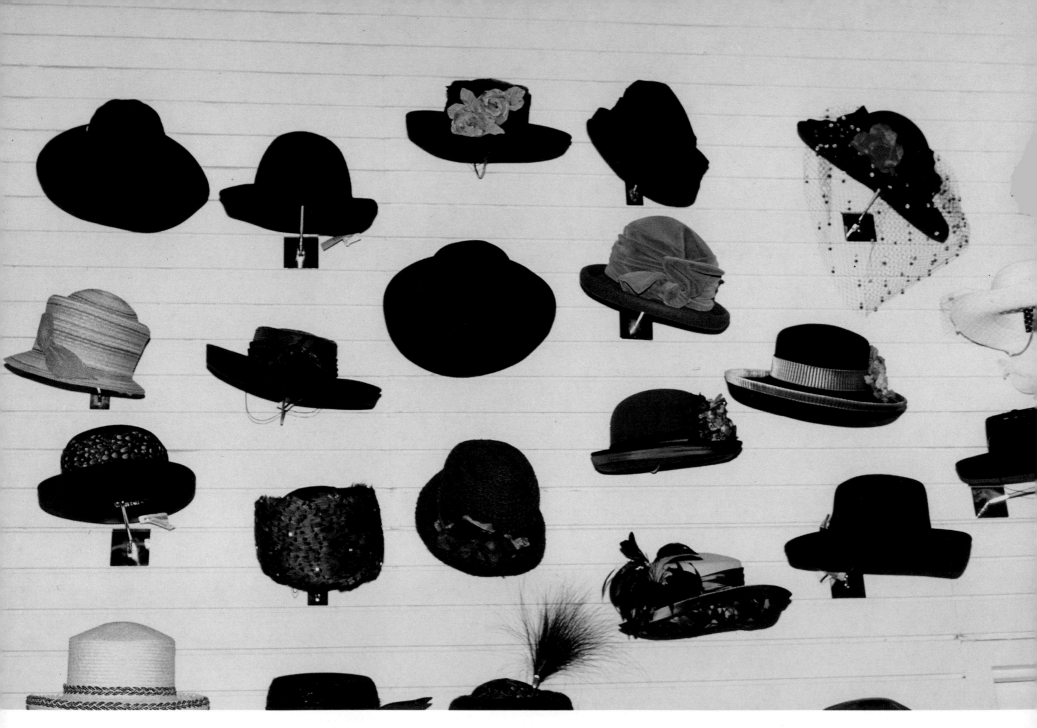

Designer hats for special occasions.

Collecting

You are best collecting what you like, not speculating on what you think may be valuable, either now or in the near future. Always collect what pleases you and you'll enjoy your collection.

If you plan to wear your hats, stay away from the very early bonnets, and fragments of bonnets. They're small and very fragile. The large, late Victorian and Edwardian straws and silks, although also fragile, can be worn if they're in good condition. The Edwardian fur felts tend to be the most durable of the early bunch, and if found unadorned, can be augmented with a feather or hatpin, if that's your preference.

The decades of the 1920s through 1950s offer many wearable choices for hat collectors. Some women collect and wear only cloches; others wear wide-brimmed natural straws.

In her book, *Hats: a stylish history and collector's guide,* Jody Shields offers a few helpful hints for evaluating a hat. Much of this is common sense. When buying an old hat, unless you're looking for a relic, condition should be top priority. In evaluating condition, weigh such factors as relative rarity of the hat, age, style, material, and designer. Learn to look carefully, whether you buy in upscale vintage shops, vintage shows, auctions, flea markets, or thrift stores. Learn to look.

The focus of *Hats* is hat collecting in America. Many of our top stores included branches in Paris or London, but this book does not include European designers. It does, however, include examples of early hats sold by "importers" and "official reproductions" made in America from French models. The subject of Paris millinery could be addressed in a future, enlarged edition. As hat collectors we prize hats by many of the American designers included in *Hats:* Lilly Daché, Hattie Carnegie, Mr. John, Erik, Irene, Laddie Northridge, Sally Victor, Don Anderson, Emme, and Frank Olive, to name a few.

You will notice as you review the descriptions in the book that many exceptional hats are not labeled. If a hat has a designer and/or store label, it is mentioned. In listing as many milliners as possible, I intended to increase the frame of reference we have as collectors, for names, styles, and periods of activity.

Bibliography

Baumgarten, Linda. *Eighteenth-Century Clothing at Williamsburg.* Williamsburg, Virginia: The Colonial Williamsburg Foundation, 1986.

Blum, Dilys E. *Ahead of Fashion: Hats of the 20th Century, Bulletin,* volume 89, number 377-78. Philadelphia: Philadelphia Museum of Art, Summer/Fall 1993,

Fairchild's Dictionary of Fashion, 2nd Edition. Edited by Charlotte Mankey Calasibetta. New York: Fairchild Publications, 1988.

Ginsburg, Madeleine. *The Hat: Trends and Traditions.* Hauppauge, New York: Barrons Educational Series, 1990.

The Imperial: A Journal For the Home. Poughkeepsie, New York: Imperial Publishing Co., August 14, 1894.

McDowell, Colin. *Hats: Status, Style And Glamour.* New York: Rizzoli International Publications, Inc., 1992.

Sears, Roebuck and Company Catalog, No. 171, Fall and Winter, 1935-36.

Sears, Roebuck and Company Catalog, No. 176, Spring and Summer, 1938.

Shields, Jody. *Hats: a stylish history and collector's guide.* New York: Clarkson N. Potter, Inc., 1991.

Tozer, Jane and Sarah Levitt. *Fabric of Society: A Century of People and Their Clothes, 1770-1870.* Carno, Powys, Wales: Laura Ashley Limited, 1983.

Weiss, Harry B. And Grace M. Weiss. *The Early Hatters of New Jersey.* Trenton, New Jersey: New Jersey Agricultural Society, 1961.

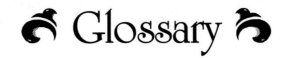 Glossary

acetate Generic term for fiber artificially made from cellulose acetate, often used for linings.

appliqué Surface pattern made by cutting out fabric or lace designs and attaching them to another fabric by means of embroidering or stitching.

baronet satin Lustrous fabric made in satin weave; popular before 1930.

beret Round, soft, brimless cap.

bonnet A close-fitting brimmed hat, tied under the chin with ribbons.

buckram Loosely woven, heavily sized fabric in a plain weave used for stiffening; similar to crinoline.

cage A large cap made of veiling which covers the head and face and may be decorated with flowers, velvet bows, etc. A wisp of veiling, a "minimal" or "whimsy" hat. Popular in the 1960s.

calash Large collapsible hood worn from 1720 to 1790 and revived from 1820 to 1839; made with hinged arches of whalebone; called calèche after the hood of a French carriage.

cartwheel A hat with an exaggerated wide brim and a low crown.

cellophane A thin, transparent film, made of acetate.

clip Half-hat mounted on a spring-metal clip, worn across the crown of the head.

cloche A tight-fitting, deep crowned hat with a narrow brim, usually worn pulled down over the eyebrows.

confections Name given to millinery decorations, ca. 1890.

cord or cording Trimming made by inserting a soft rope-like cord into a strip of bias-cut fabric.

cowboy hat A wide-brimmed felt hat with a tall creased or uncreased crown and a brim rolled up on the sides and dipped in front; ten gallon hat, Stetson, western hat.

designer The artist who creates the hats.

doll hat A miniature or doll sized hat, usually worn over the forehead and secured with round elastic.

Dunstable The Dunstable way, a road running from London to the municipal borough of Dunstable, Bedfordshire, England, known for its straightness; hence the adjective meaning plain, direct, and straight. This term used in the description "in Betsy Metcalf's own hand[writing]" very likely refers to the Dunstable way.

duvetyne A smooth, lustrous, velvety fabric that has a napped surface which obscures the twill weave.

Empress Eugénie A 1930s small hat, pitched forward to one side of the face, based on a hat style worn by Empress Eugénie, wife of Napoleon III (1852-1870).

faille Fabric with a flat-ribbed effect running fillingwise; flatter and less pronounced than grosgrain.

fedora A hat with a medium sized brim, high crown, and a crease from front to back.

fur felt Material that includes wool in combination with such fur fibers as llama, vicuña, beaver, or rabbit.

generic A less expensive version of a designer original hat, lacking the designer label; "knock-off," "no-brand" substitute.

grosgrain Ribbon with rib more rounded than faille that is made with several filling yarns used together. Made originally in silk, now made mostly with rayon or acetate warp and cotton or rayon filling.

helmet A close-fitting cap with sides extending over the ears.

hood Soft, draped hat, may extend to the shoulders.

horsehair Hair fiber from the mane and tail of a horse; may be used in combination with mohair, linen or cotton to achieve an open-work effect.; crin is the French term.

importers Buyers, such as John Wanamaker, that regularly imported European, especially French hats for the American market.

jersey Classification of knitted fabrics that are knitted in a plain stitch without a distinct rib.

Leghorn English name for Livorno, Italy, known for its high quality straw; type of straw.

millinery Women's head coverings, specifically hats, bonnets, caps, hoods, and veils.

mohair Hair of the angora goat; may be mixed with other fibers.

mushroom A hat with a deep, usually puffed crown , and a medium brim.

nylon Generic term for an artificial fiber made of a long chair of synthetic polyamides extracted from coal and petroleum.

official reproduction A hat copied from a French model with the milliner's permission; copies were generally less expensive than the originals.

ombre dye Dyeing flowers in related tones of monochromatic, or same color, shading.

open-crown, halo A wide-brimmed hat without a crown.

peau de soie Heavyweight satin with a fine filling ribbed effect on the reverse side, made of silk or synthetic fibers, from the French meaning "skin of silk."

Panama Hat made of very fine straw of the jipijapa plant, handwoven in Ecuador.

picture hat A hat with a large, face-framing brim.

pile Loops or other yarns which stand erect on fabric to form all, or part, of the fabric surface.

pillbox Classic round, brimless hat sometimes worn forward on the head; introduced in the 1920s and worn since with slight variations.

poke bonnet Bonnet of the 19th century, made with a wide brim slanting forward from a small crown to frame and shadow the face.

pompons Round ball of cut ends of yarn used as trimming; hair or cap ornament composed of feathers; tinsel, etc.

princess style A small skullcap, similar to the clip hat, often made of silk, or lace, and edged in pearls. Also known as the Juliet cap. Made famous by Princess Grace of Monaco.

rayon Fiber derived from trees, cotton, and woody plants, shiny and lustrous, but less expensive than silk.

Romandi Italian synthetic straw, made with polypropylene (a substance resembling polyethylene or polyisobutylene used in making fibers, films, and molded products).

rosette Ornament arranged like a rose; usually ribbon arranged in standing loops or flattened into a formal pattern.

ruching Trim that is pleated and stitched so that it ruffles on both sides.

silk Fiber from the cocoon of the silkworm; sheer, smooth, and luxurious.

slouch A hat with a flexible brim, which may be turned down in front; also known as the Garbo hat.

smock-stitch or smoking Decorative needlework used to hold gathered cloth together; the stitches catch alternate folds in elaborate honeycombed designs.

snap-brim A hat with a brim that may be worn at several different angles.

snood A woven or knotted net, worn to cover or contain the hair.

Stetson John B. Stetson, Philadelphia; trade name synonymous with the western, cowboy hat; or ten-gallon hat.

taffeta Term used for a classification of crisp fabrics with a fine, smooth surface; originally made in silk, now made in synthetic fibers.

tam-ó-shanter A wide, flat beret, with a tight headband; originally Scottish.

tea hat Similar to a pillbox in design; usually made of lace or silk for semiformal wear.

toque A small, close-fitting, brimless cap.

tricorne 19th century term for "cocked hat" turned up to form three equidistant peaks with one peak in front; first worn by men during the 17th century.

tulle Fine sheer net fabric made of silk, nylon, or rayon with hexagonal holes.

turban A head-dress or scarf wound directly around the head or around a cap.

velour Soft velvety thick pile fabric used for good quality hats; from French velours.

Price Reference

If it's difficult to date old hats, it's almost impossible to price them. Unlike many other collectibles, you will never find two exactly alike. Condition, age, designer label versus no label at all, style, and material all affect price. If a hat is in its original box, and the box is in good condition, a collector should expect to pay more. If a hat is extremely rare, for example a miniature velvet Stetson in its original holiday box, the seller can name the price!

My older son and I recently attended an antiques show together. My son, who collects Native American pottery and baskets, was discussing the merits of an early basket with one of the show's dealers, and after much description of the basket in question, my son remarked, "I guess it's really priceless."

"No," the dealer said, "it has a price." So that's how we have to look at hats. Some are very special and very rare, and the price is very likely to be high. Hats that are not as rare are likely to be priced lower.

Highest prices for early hats are paid for those with excellent provenance, as to ownership and descent, and exact age. Fragments of early hats, because of their age, are always of interest to museums and collectors. Here, again, provenance raises the price. The fragments or relics in poor condition, without any provenance, should cost relatively little ($50-100). The early fur felt hats, because they are sparsely decorated and more readily available, are also less expensive. The 1890s is a very collectible period, therefore prices tend to be high. From 1920-1960, designer hats tend to be considerably more expensive than generics or those without labels.

Regional variations and selling venue dramatically affect hat prices. Prices are not given when such information is unavailable or inappropriate, such as museum collections. Prices are unavailable for custom and contemporary millinery.

On the cover		1700-2500		top right	75-125	Page 30	left	95-115		right	45-60
Page 6		NPA		bottom right	60-75		right	85-100	Page 42	left	65-85
Page 7		50-100	Page 19	top left	95-150	Page 31	left	85-110		top right	85-110
Page 8	top left	50-100		bottom left	175-250		right	65-85		bottom right	75-95
	bottom right	50-75		right	60-75	Page 32	left	45-60	Page 43	left	65-85
Page 9	left	350-400	Page 20	left	65-85		top right	45-60		right	45-60
	top right	300-375		right	75-95		bottom right	40-55	Page 44	left	65-85
Page 10	left	300-350	Page 21	top left	NPA	Page 33	right	175-210	Page 45	right	50-65
	right	NPA		bottom left	75-100	Page 34	left	350-425	Page 46	left	65-80
Page 11	top left	300-350		right	40-60		top right	175-210		right	45-60
	top right	325-375	Page 22	left	110-150		bottom right	125-150	Page 47	left	65-85
	bottom	400-450		right	65-85	Page 35	top left	175-210		right	50-65
Page 12	top left	350-375	Page 23	top left	65-85		bottom left	NPA	Page 48	left	50-65
	top right	NPA		bottom left	50-70		right	200-225		right	40-60
	bottom left	325-375		right	55-75	Page 36	left	50-65	Page 49	left	65-80
Page 13	top left, with basket	750-1000	Page 24	left	85-125		center	85-110		right	65-80
	right	NPA		top right	75-95		right	75-95	Page 50	left	175-250
Page 14	top left	NPA		bottom right	NPA	Page 37	left	95-120	Page 51	left	65-80
	right,	NPA	Page 25	left	65-85		center	75-95		right	45-60
Page 15	left	95-150		right	50-70		right	95-120	Page 52	left	45-60
	right	75-125	Page 26	left	50-75	Page 38	left	50-65		right	40-55
Page 16	left	275-350		top right	50-75		right	NPA	Page 53	left	65-80
	top right	200-250		bottom right	85-125	Page 39	left	45-65		right	55-75
	bottom right	175-225	Page 27	left	35-50		right	35-55	Page 54	left	55-75
Page 17	left	65-85		right	90-110	Page 40	left	65-85		right	60-75
	center	50-75	Page 28	top left	NPA		top right	45-60	Page 55	top left	50-65
	right	50-75		bottom right	45-60		bottom left	65-85		bottom left	45-60
Page 18	left	45-60	Page 29	on model	65-85	Page 41	left	45-60		right (on model)	65-80

Page	Location	Value
Page 56	left	45-55
	top left	65-80
	bottom left	45-55
Page 57	top left	40-50
	bottom left	65-80
	right (on model)	90-110
Page 58	top left	90-110
	top right	65-85
	bottom right	45-60
Page 59	top left	40-50
	bottom left	65-80
	right	NPA
Page 60	top left	45-60
	bottom left	85-110
	top right	75-90
	bottom right	NPA
Page 61	top left	50-65
	bottom left	40-50
	right	NPA
Page 62	left	45-65
	top right	55-75
	bottom right	65-85
Page 63	left	NPA
	right	65-85
Page 64	left	65-85
	top right	55-75
	bottom right	40-50
Page 65	right	100-125
Page 66	left	NPA
	right	295-350
Page 67	top left	NPA
	bottom left	NPA
	right	NPA
Page 68	left	75-90
	top right	65-85
	bottom right	85-100
Page 69	right	NPA
Page 70	full page	NPA
Page 71	top left	NPA
	bottom left	NPA
	right	150-175
Page 72	left	165-225
	top right	65-85
	bottom right	70-95
Page 73	top left	150-185
	bottom left	55-75
	right	65-85
Page 74	left	110-125
	right	150-185

Page	Location	Value
Page 75	top left	140-175
	bottom left	NPA
	right	NPA
Page 76	left	50-65
	right (on model)	75-95
Page 77	top left	60-75
	bottom left	55-70
	right	75-95
Page 78	left	65-85
	top right	185-250
	bottom right	60-75
Page 79	top left	35-40
	bottom left	65-80
	right	45-55
Page 80	top left	40-50
	bottom left	85-110
	right	45-55
Page 81	left	75-90
	right	55-75
Page 82	left	NPA
Page 83	left	NPA
	right	NPA
Page 84	left	325-400
	center	NPA
	right	150-175
Page 85	left	500-625
	right	250-325
Page 86	left (as is)	150-225
	top right	NPA
	bottom right	NPA
Page 87	top left	175-225
	bottom left	175-225
	center	150-175
	right	250-325
Page 88	left	95-115
	top right	NPA
	bottom right	NPA
Page 89	top left	95-115
	bottom left	110-125
	right	125-150
Page 90	left	60-75
	top right	60-75
	bottom right	150-225
Page 91	top left	75-95
	bottom left	45-55
	right	95-110
Page 92	top left	65-85
	bottom left	45-55
	top right	75-95

Page	Location	Value
	bottom right	NPA
Page 93	right	350-425
Page 94	left	275-325
	top right	60-75
	bottom right	NPA
Page 95	top left	80-95
	bottom left	85-110
	right	85-110
Page 96	left	95-125
	top right	65-85
	bottom left (w/box)	95-150
Page 97	top left	65-85
	top right	75-95
	bottom right	40-50
Page 98	left (on model)	85-110
	right	85-110
Page 99	left	350-500
	top right	250-375
	bottom right	110-150
Page 100	top left	45-55
	bottom left	65-85
	top right	65-85
	bottom right	45-55
Page 101	top left	95-125
	bottom left	85-110
	right	45-55
Page 102	left	85-110
	top right	50-65
	bottom right	50-65
Page 103	left	NPA
	top right	65-85
	bottom right	45-55
Page 104	top left	65-85
	bottom left	85-110
	top right	45-55
	bottom right	45-65
Page 105	top left	55-65
	bottom left	85-110
	right	65-85
Page 106	top left	55-65
	bottom left	60-70
	right	35-45
Page 107	left and right	175-225
Page 108	left	85-110
	right	75-95
Page 109	right	45-60
Page 110	left	NPA
	top right	65-85
	bottom right	85-110

Page	Location	Value
Page 111	left	NPA
	right (on model)	65-85
Page 112	top left	50-65
	bottom left	50-65
	right	NPA
Page 113	top left	50-65
	bottom left	40-65
	top right	40-55
	bottom right	50-60
Page 114	left	40-50
	right	50-60
Page 115	left	40-50
	right	50-65
Page 116	top left	35-45
	bottom left	35-45
	right	50-60
Page 117	left	50-65
	center	60-75
	right	60-75
Page 118	left	NPA
	top right	35-40
	bottom right	35-45
Page 119	left	35-45
	center	NPA
	right	NPA
Page 120	left	-110
	bottom right	150-200
Page 121	top left	20-30 each
	bottom left	50-65
	right	50-65
Page 122	left	65-85
	top right	65-85
	bottom right	45-55
Page 123	top left	65-75
	bottom left	55-65
	right	50-65
Page 124	left	50-75
	top right	50-75
	bottom right	45-55
Page 125	top left	85-110
	bottom left	75-95
	right	60-75
Page 126	top left	50-65
	top right	50-65
	bottom right	65-75
Page 127	top left	NPA
	bottom left	65-75
	top right	55-65

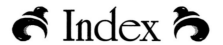 Index

Some of the labels shown with the Index are on hats not included in this book.

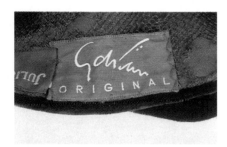

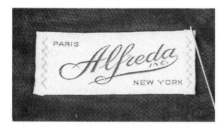

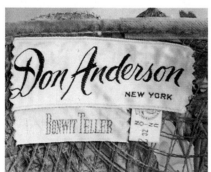

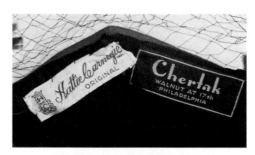

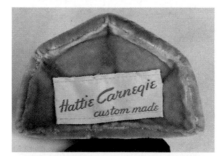

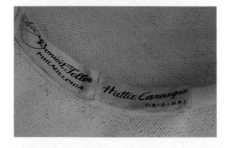

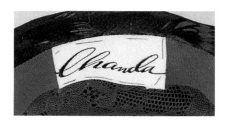

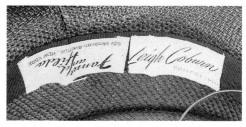

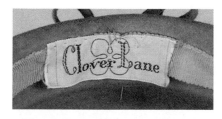

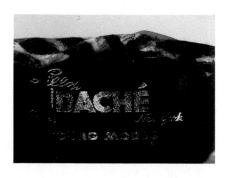

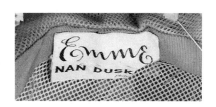

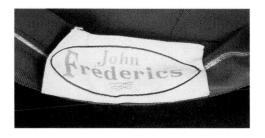

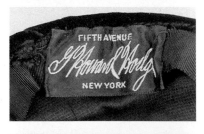

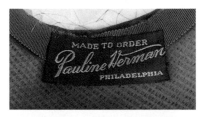

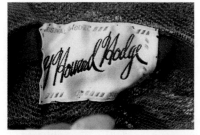

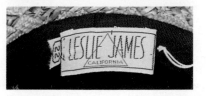

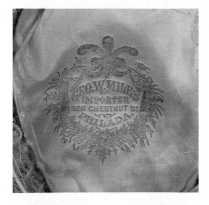

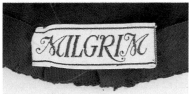

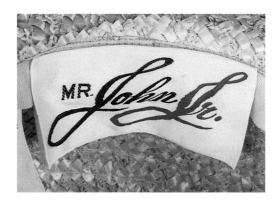

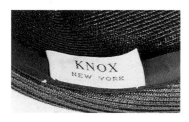

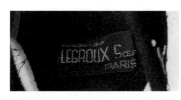

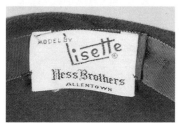

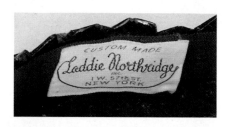

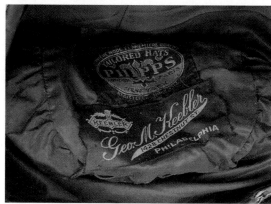

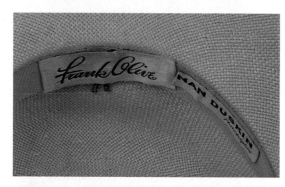

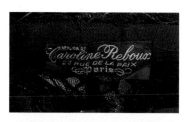

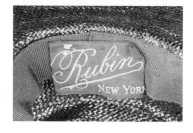

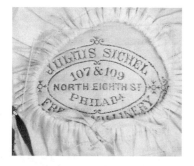

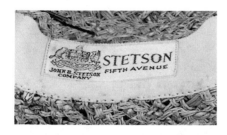

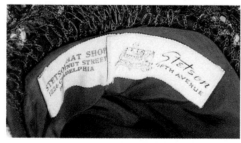

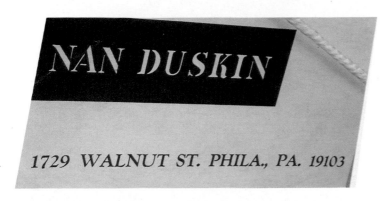

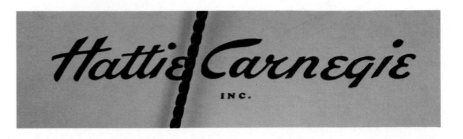

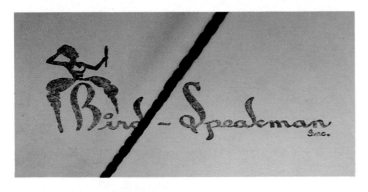

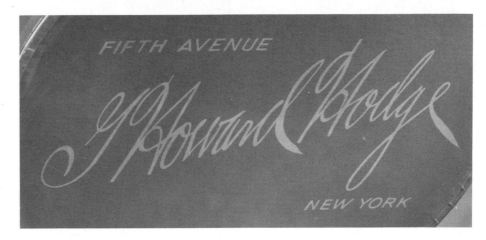

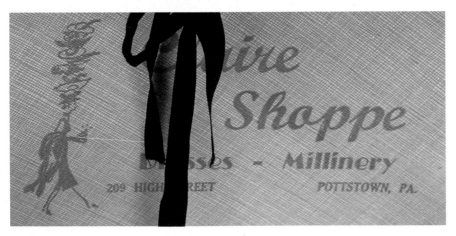

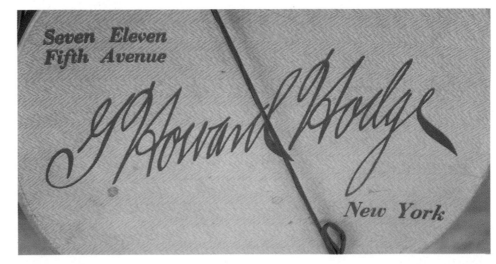